P9-DCI-858

The Women's Guide to Health

This book was carefully researched. However, all information is supplied without liability. Neither the authors nor the publisher will be liable for possible disadvantages or damages resulting from this book.

JEFF GALLOWAY
RUTH PARKER
CARMEN PATRICK MOHAN

THE WOMEN'S GUIDE
TO HEALTH

RUN WALK RUN ,
EAT RIGHT,
AND FEEL BETTER

Meyer & Meyer Sport

British Library Cataloguing in Publication Data
A catalogue record for this book is available from the British Library

Women's Guide to Health: Run Walk Run, Eat Right, and Feel Better
Maidenhead: Meyer & Meyer Sport (UK) Ltd., 2018
ISBN 978-1-78255-123-2

All rights reserved, especially the right to copy and distribute, including the translation rights.
No part of this work may be reproduced—including by photocopy, microfilm or any other means—
processed, stored electronically, copied or distributed in any form whatsoever without the written
permission of the publisher.

© 2018 by Meyer & Meyer Sport (UK) Ltd.
Aachen, Auckland, Beirut, Budapest, Cairo, Cape Town, Dubai, Hägendorf,
Indianapolis, Maidenhead, Singapore, Sydney, Tehran, Vienna

 Member of the World Sport Publishers' Association (WSPA)

Printed by C-M Books, Ann Arbor, MI, USA
ISBN 978-1-78255-123-2
E-Mail: info@m-m-sports.com
www.m-m-sports.com

CONTENTS

Medical Disclaimer: The contents of this book are not intended nor implied to be relied on for medical diagnosis, care or treatment concerning any individual. Under no circumstances, will this book create a physician-patient relationship, nor does it constitute engagement in the practice of medicine or the provision of any health care service to an individual patient. This book should not be used as a substitute for professional diagnosis and treatment, and readers should consult a healthcare provider before making any healthcare decisions or for guidance about medical conditions. The authors of this book expressly disclaim responsibility, and shall have no liability, for any damages, loss, injury, or liability whatsoever suffered as a result of a reader's reliance on the information contained in this book.

Acknowledgments

Medicine and Public Health Advisory Board

Barbara Galloway – Galloway Productions

Rose Martinez, ScD – Director, Board on Population Health and Public Health Practice Health and Medicine Division; The National Academies of Sciences, Engineering, and Medicine

James Roberson, MD – Professor and Chairman, Department of Orthopedics; Emory University School of Medicine; Past President of the Society of Joint Surgeons

Larry Sperling, MD – Professor of Medicine (Cardiology); Emory University School of Medicine; President, American Society of Preventive Cardiology

Guillermo Umpierrez, MD – Professor of Medicine; Director of Diabetes, Grady Health System; Emory University School of Medicine; National Board of Directors of American Diabetes Association

Photography Credit

Nikki Strayhorn
Brennan Galloway

INTRODUCTION

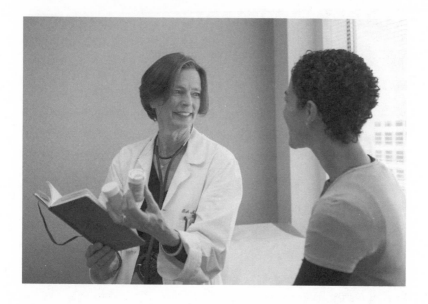

What we all want is to feel good in our own skin. After all, isn't that what health is about? We want to feel connected to those we love most. We want to have the emotional resilience needed to cope with life's challenges, and to have a positive attitude that helps us feel grateful and enjoy living. To do this, we need healthy bodies, minds, and spirits. The authors of this guide believe that when the body gets into motion, it unlocks parts of the mind and spirit that are a reservoir of energy and goodness. This indescribably wonderful source of energy is amplified when we run-walk-run with others. Our physical bodies function at their highest level when they are nourished by healthy foods. Chances are you're not eating as well or being as active as you'd like to be— hardly anyone is. That's why we got together to write this guide to the HER Prescriptions™ Program (www.HERprescriptions.com). HER stands for **h**ealthy **e**ating and **r**un-walking.

This book guides you through a proven sequence of actions you can take over the next 30 weeks to change your habits and start a path to feeling better, more energetic, and more connected to others. Think of this book as an action guide that combines the knowledge and experience of a highly respected Run-Walk coach with real world advice from two primary care medical doctors. All three of us have used what we present here in our own lives, the lives of our families, and the lives of thousands of women we have coached or seen as patients. We know it works.

Every day, each of us can take control over our exercise, our eating, and our attitude by having specific cognitive strategies. Having a specific strategy is key for motivation. Our step-by-step process gives you control and focus—it can empower you to make many positive changes in your life. Your health and the health of your family and community ALL benefit.

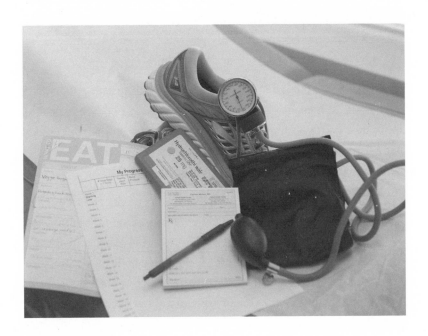

The first chapter focuses on journaling and teaches you how and what to record about your health. You learn to log the essentials for health: sleep, exercise, quality of food, and meals. You also learn how to track and record the health numbers of interest to you. You will create a starting line for yourself as you begin recording and envision the finish line.

Chapter 2 helps guide you to a successful start. We cover common health considerations for women beginning the HER Prescription program.

In chapter 3, we help you choose the HER Prescription that is right for you. We cover the specifics of three different training program options: Rx Run-Walk Get Started, Rx Run-Walk Keep Going, and Rx Run-Walk Burn Fat. Each Rx Run-Walk has a 30-week training program proven to help you reach the fully prescribed dose.

To reach your health goals, your Rx Run-Walk should be combined with a prescription about what you eat. We call this your Rx Eat. Your prescribed Rx Eat (chapter 4) tells you what to eat, how often to eat, and how to record this in your health journal.

In chapter 5, we set you up for success with healthy eating. You learn why sleep is fundamental to health and helping us choose healthy foods. We give you tools for meal planning, grocery shopping, and perfect score recipes that fit with your Rx Eat. We also offer tips to address common challenges while following your Rx Eat.

In chapter 6, we rely on best available medical evidence to tell you how your HER Prescriptions can help you meet specific health goals. We take a look at how the prescribed Rx Run-Walk and Rx Eat improve common health conditions including high blood pressure, high cholesterol or lipids (fat in the blood), heart disease, osteoarthritis (aching bones or joints), breathing difficulties such as asthma or COPD, diabetes, anxiety, and depression. For some women, these health conditions are related to excess weight. That's why, throughout the book, we provide specific details for finding your healthy weight. Those seeking to lose weight are coached up to the 30-week, fully prescribed dose of Rx Run-Walk and Rx Eat and asked to maintain it for at least 3 months. On the weight loss track, you can expect to lose about 0.5 to 1lbs weekly (20 to 50 pounds over 1 year) and feel a whole lot better!

For those who have been hospitalized with medical conditions such as a heart attack (myocardial infarction), heart rhythm problems, cancer, stroke, or lung disease, we strongly recommend you discuss and follow a specific rehabilitation program under the supervision of your doctor. For the millions who have not been hospitalized but have been diagnosed with a chronic condition or illness for which you see a primary care provider, this book uses medical evidence, quality meal plans, and a well-established training program's approach to provide the fundamentals you need to know to improve your health.

Use this book as an action guide and follow it step by step. All the charts, tables, and journal pages can be found on our website, www.HERprescriptions.com. Download them, print them out, and tape them to your fridge. Like prescriptions for medicines, these prescriptions only work if you take them regularly and carefully follow the instructions.

Are you ready? Let's get started. Look forward to feeling better, happier, and more alive and engaged in your everyday life as you move through this. It's an amazing feeling and worth your time and dedication. You can do it…and will be so glad you did!

CHAPTER 1
JOURNAL

Your journal will inspire you and will be a pivotal part of your success in reaching your health goals!

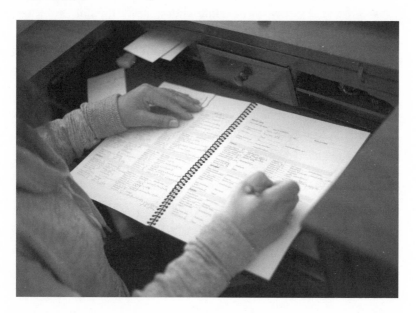

Improving your health depends on becoming an expert on your own mind, body, and spirit. The key to becoming such an expert is being rigid about organization, note taking and record keeping, and time for personal reflection. Women who are most successful in achieving their health goals have cultivated the habit of recording four variables each day: sleep, exercise, food, and health numbers. We believe the reason these women are so successful in achieving their health goals relates to their habit of keeping a health journal that harnesses focus, attention, motivation, and insight. A journal is not only essential for gaining knowledge about yourself. The act of gathering the data and recording in your journal is the most important action you can take because it activates your problem-solving brain, giving you control over your daily activities and food choices. This puts you in command of each area of your health, every day.

The health journal prompts you to record daily and reflect weekly. Each day has the following four parts: sleep metrics, exercise matters, food score, and meal log. In addition, there is a three-part weekly report card to help you summarize progress, chart important health numbers, and hone in on what works for you.

The health journal is designed to help you navigate meaningful conversations with your doctor. Sharing your journal with your doctor helps in the following ways:

- ✓ Your doctor reviews information you feel is important to your health and well-being.

- ✓ Your doctor has better numbers upon which to base medical decisions.

- ✓ You are an active partner with your doctor in recognizing trends and patterns related to how you feel.

Getting Started: How to Create Your Own Starting Line Using the Health Journal

Where are you starting from? Knowing this will help you develop the right expectations of yourself and others. It will also give you a better understanding of your progress when you look back over the weeks and months.

What you will need:

- a digital scale that can also measure body fat composition

- a flexible tape measure

- a pedometer or other device that counts steps such as a smart phone or watch

- commitment to filling out the health journal for 7 consecutive days starting with Monday

Your starting line consists of the following measurements:

1. Body weight

2. Body fat composition

3. Waist circumference

AND

4. One week of recording sleep metrics

AND

5. One week of exercise matters

AND

6. One week of recording everything you eat

Step 1

Locate the Starting Line Journal Pages in the appendix. Tear them out and copy them (or use the originals). Look for the table shown on the following page.

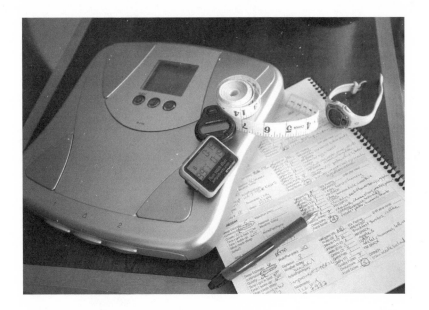

SLEEP METRICS	EXERCISE MATTERS	MEALS
Monday		
Sleep estimate:_____ continuous/uninterrupted Quality: _____ Time I got in bed: _____ Time I woke up: _____	Run-walk (min): _____ Steps: _____	Breakfast AM snack Lunch PM snack Dinner
Tuesday		
Sleep estimate:_____ continuous/uninterrupted Quality: _____ Time I got in bed: _____ Time I woke up: _____	Run-walk (min): _____ Steps: _____	Breakfast AM snack Lunch PM snack Dinner
Wednesday		
Sleep estimate:_____ continuous/uninterrupted Quality: _____ Time I got in bed: _____ Time I woke up: _____	Run-walk (min): _____ Steps: _____	Breakfast AM snack Lunch PM snack Dinner
Thursday		
Sleep estimate:_____ continuous/uninterrupted Quality: _____ Time I got in bed: _____ Time I woke up: _____	Run-walk (min): _____ Steps: _____	Breakfast AM snack Lunch PM snack Dinner

Step 2

Record your starting body weight and body fat composition. Starting on Monday morning, get up, pee, and get onto the digital scale. Weigh yourself in the nude before taking a shower, then record it. Record

Starting Line Report Card

HEALTH NUMBERS		REFLECTIONS
Weight: _____		I feel…
Waist: _____		
Body fat % _____		
BP: _____ / _____		What works well for me?

Friday

Sleep estimate:_____ continuous/uninterrupted	Run-walk (min): _____	Breakfast
	Steps: _____	AM snack
Quality: _____		Lunch
Time I got in bed: _____		PM snack
Time I woke up: _____		Dinner

Saturday

Sleep estimate:_____ continuous/uninterrupted	Run-walk (min): _____	Breakfast
	Steps: _____	AM snack
Quality: _____		Lunch
Time I got in bed: _____		PM snack
Time I woke up: _____		Dinner

Sunday

Sleep estimate:_____ continuous/uninterrupted	Run-walk (min): _____	Breakfast
	Steps: _____	AM snack
Quality: _____		Lunch
Time I got in bed: _____		PM snack
Time I woke up: _____		Dinner

your body fat composition percentage, a number you get from your digital scale.

Reasons for knowing your starting body weight are self-explanatory, but why should you also know your body fat composition? Two reasons. First, body weight fluctuates. From day to day, the amount of water our bodies hold changes our weight without giving us much information that pertains to health. Second, in the first few weeks and months, your weight might not change at all. This is because as you exercise, your muscles will strengthen and grow. Muscles weigh more than fat, so as you lose fat, you might not lose weight. Nevertheless, you'll be healthier than you were before you started. One

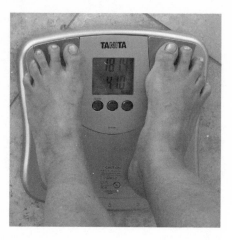

way to measure this healthy trend is by checking to see if your body fat composition goes down. Health, not weight loss, is the real goal here.

Step 3

Before you put on any clothing, measure your waist circumference. To do this correctly, stand up straight. Your waist is located above your belly button and below your rib cage. Hold the end of the tape measure just above your belly button and bring it around your waist to the

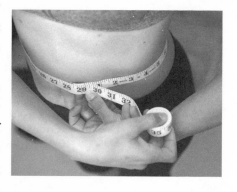

front. Be sure to place the tape measure directly on your skin, snugly but without digging into it. The measuring tape should be parallel to the floor. Don't try to suck your gut in! Look at the place on the tape where the zero end meets the other end of the tape measure. The location of this meeting point is your waist measurement (Resource: WikiHow, www.wikihow.com/Measure-Your-Waist).

Step 4

Record the total time you spend walking or running. Record the number of steps you took each day.

Step 5

Start estimating how much you sleep. Note whether sleep was interrupted. Describe sleep quality as poor, fair, or good. Note the time you get into bed and the time you wake up.

Step 6

Write down everything you eat and drink. Note the approximate time of day. For now, don't worry about trying to count calories, but do try to estimate your portion sizes.

Your First Week: How to Begin and Continue

In order to get the most accurate record for your starting line, you'll have to keep the journal with you at all times. It should be on your night stand at night and in your purse or briefcase if you go out. If you forget to record something, note it down later in the correct place as best as you can and as soon as you can. Consider setting an alarm or even several alarms to help you remember to write down your meals and snacks. At the end of every day, review the entry and plug any holes you find.

Keep Going With Journaling for Healthy Weight

As you make your way through this book, we will make recommendations for increasing the level of detail in your journal. Here are some overarching suggestions:

✓ Weigh yourself once weekly at most. Do this in the morning. Get up, pee, and weigh yourself in the nude (before taking a shower), and then record your body weight and composition. Weighing yourself more than once per week is probably a waste of time. Since it takes about one to two weeks to lose 0.5 to 1 pound of fat, you are not likely to see meaningful changes in your weight in less than one week's time.

✓ Reflect on daily, weekly, and monthly entries to help you identify the most useful strategies for weight loss over time.

✓ Record the health metrics or numbers of interest to you. Not every number will fit with your needs. For example, fasting blood sugar, resting heart rate, and blood pressure are not necessarily something you need to track if you don't have health conditions that relate to these. In chapter 6, we will teach you more about medical conditions and make recommendations for additional health numbers which might be important for you to measure and record in your journal.

✓ Your journal should help keep you on track and help you identify specific areas where you need to improve so that you can reach your health goals. For this reason, we recommend you total and chart your numbers week by week. At the end of each week, add summary information to the Week Log found in the appendix. See pages 24 and 25 for a sample Week Log.

Cross out any column you do not intend to record. For example, if you do not have a glucometer (a machine for checking blood sugar) you will not be recording in the fasting blood sugar column.

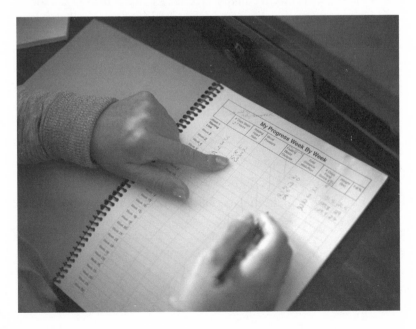

Know Where You're Going: How to Create a Finish Line

When it comes to healthy habits like exercise and eating, these are lifelong endeavors that never finish. If you run-walk 150 minutes per week and eat a balanced diet like the one we advocate for in this book, you can maintain a healthy weight throughout your life.

However, it seems like losing weight is a never-ending goal on the list of New Year's resolutions. Our view is that this fixation with weight loss is just not healthy for anyone. Instead, in this book, we give you evidence-based prescriptions to run-walk, eat right, and feel better. We give you tools to learn about yourself in the level of detail needed to make choices that meet your health goals and allow you to have meaningful conversations with your doctor.

If your goal is to treat a medical condition related to excess weight (the focus of chapter 6), we recommend collaborating with your doctor to decide on a weight loss finish line that's right for you. Here's how to have a meaningful conversation with your doctor about weight loss:

- ✓ Schedule a visit with your doctor specifically to discuss weight loss without any other concern on your agenda. You want the focus of the visit to be obtaining professional advice about weight loss.

- ✓ When the assistant checks your blood pressure, heart rate, weight, and blood glucose (if applicable), record the numbers in your health journal and compare them to those at home for accuracy.

- ✓ Tell your doctor you are looking to lose weight and why.

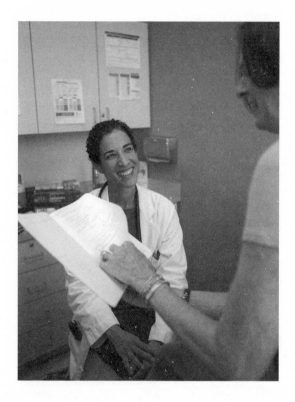

✓ Ask your doctor about which of your medical conditions might be helped by weight loss.

✓ Ask your doctor how much weight you need to lose to help treat your medical condition.

✓ Show your doctor the Rx Run-Walk (chapter 3) and Rx Eat (chapter 4) you plan to follow and ask if any modifications are recommended.

✓ If you have remaining questions or concerns, ask for a referral to a nutritionist.

My Progress Week By Week

	Number of days slept ≥7 hours	Resting heart rate	Blood pressure	Fasting blood glucose	Total distance run-walk	Number of days with a food score ≥6	Weight (lbs)	Fat %
Starting line								
Week 1								
Week 2								
Week 3								
Week 4								
Week 5								
Week 6								
Week 7								
Week 8								
Week 9								
Week 10								
Week 11								
Week 12								
Week 13								

Week 14	Week 15	Week 16	Week 17	Week 18	Week 19	Week 20	Week 21	Week 22	Week 23	Week 24	Week 25	Week 26	Week 27	Week 28	Week 29	Week 30

Your weight loss finish line should be informed by the above conversation with your doctor. Know that evidence shows moderate weight loss (defined as losing 5 to 10% of your baseline weight) is associated with meaningful improvement in health risk factors. At one year, people who lose 8.6% of their baseline weight have significant decreases in their blood pressure, decreased triglycerides (fat in the blood), and improved diabetes control. Larger weight loss means larger improvements (NEJM, DM Prevention Trial).

We advocate choosing a weight loss goal for the year that is no more than about 10% of your current body weight. For example, if you weigh 200lbs, your weight loss goal should be 20lbs or less in 1 year; that's about 0.5 lbs per week not including holidays. That's an ambitious goal. A good goal. A goal that is likely to improve health problems related to excess weight such as those we discuss in chapter 6.

Don't cross your personal finish line only to return to old habits. In terms of achieving and then maintaining good health, there is a finish line to weight loss. But there's no finishing the Rx Run-Walk and Rx Eat required to maintain good health or a healthy weight.

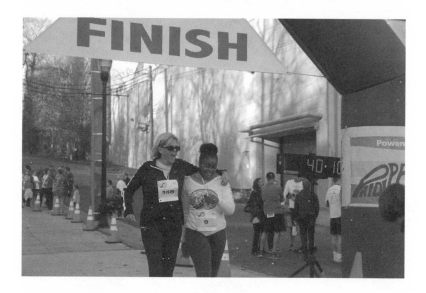

CHAPTER 2
SET YOURSELF
UP FOR
SUCCESS WITH
RX RUN/WALK

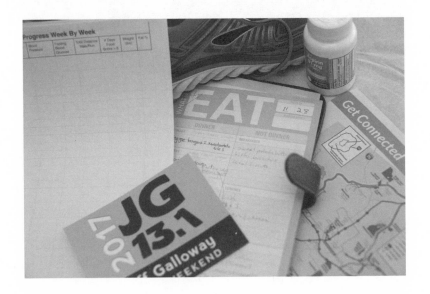

Shoes

The primary investment is usually less than $110 and more than $75. Most women who follow Rx Run-Walk wisely decide to spend a little time and money on a good running shoe. After all, shoes are the only real equipment needed. The right shoe can make running easier and reduce blisters, foot fatigue, and injuries. Because there are so many different brands with many different models, shoe shopping can be confusing. The best advice is to get the best advice. Going to a good running store, staffed by helpful and knowledgeable runners, can cut the time required and can usually lead you to a better shoe choice than you would find for yourself. A knowledgeable shoe store staff person can usually notice how your foot functions. They will watch you walk and run. This is a skill gained through the experience of fitting thousands of feet and comparing notes with other staff members who are even more experienced. Find a specialty running store near you by typing "running store" followed by your zip code into the web search engine of your choice.

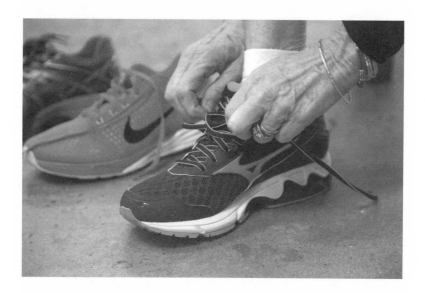

Here are some tips for your trip to the running store:

- Ask around for the best running store. You want one that has a reputation for spending time with each customer to find a shoe that will best match the shape and function of the foot.

- Your foot tends to swell during the day so it's best to get your shoes fitted after noontime.

- Bring with you the most worn pair of walking or running shoes you own.

- Be prepared to spend at least 45 minutes in the store. Quality stores are often busy, and quality fitting takes time.

- Give feedback. As you work with the person in the store, you need to give feedback as to how the shoe fits and feels. You want the shoe to protect your foot while allowing the foot to go through a natural walking and running motion for you. Tell the staff person if there are pressure points or pains or if it just doesn't feel right.

- Expensive shoes are often not the best for you. You cannot assume that higher price will buy you extra protection or more miles. At the price of some of the shoes, you might expect that they will do the running for you. They won't.

- Go by fit and not the size noted on the box of the shoe. Most runners wear a running shoe that is about two sizes larger than their street shoe. For example, Carmen wears a size 8 dress shoe but does her Rx Run-Walk in a size 10 running shoe. Be open to getting the best fit regardless of what size you see on the running shoe box.

- Try shoes on while wearing the socks you plan to use during Rx Run-Walk. Consider investing in a pair or two of running socks.

Clothing

The most important factor in choosing your Rx Run-Walk clothing is comfort. In summer, you want to wear light, cool clothing. During cold weather, layers are the best strategy. You don't have to have the latest techno-garments to run-walk. On most days, an old pair of shorts and a t-shirt are fine. As you follow your Rx Run-Walk, you will find

Clothing Thermometer

Temperature	What to Wear
14°C or 60°F and above	Tank top or singlet, shorts, socks
9 to 13°C or 50 to 59°F	T-shirt, shorts, socks
5 to 8°C or 40 to 49°F	Long-sleeve light-weight shirt, shorts or tights (or nylon long pants), socks, mittens or gloves
0 to 4°C or 30 to 39°F	Long-sleeve medium-weight shirt, another t-shirt, tights, shorts, socks, mittens or gloves, hat covering the ears
-4 to -1°C or 20 to 29°F	Long-sleeve medium-weight shirt, t-shirt or vest, tights, shorts, thick socks, mittens or gloves, hat covering the ears heavy-weight shirt, tights, shorts, nylon wind suit (top and pants), thick socks, thick mittens, hat covering the ears
-8 to -5°C or 10 to 19°F	Long-sleeve medium-weight shirt, heavy-weight shirt, tights, shorts, nylon wind suit (top and pants), thick socks, thick mittens, hat covering the ears
-12 to -9°C or 0 to 9°F	Two long-sleeve medium- or heavy-weight shirts, thick tights, thick underwear, medium-to-heavy warm-up, gloves, thick mittens, ski mask, hat covering the ears, Vaseline covering any exposed skin
-18 to -13°C or -15°F	Two long-sleeve heavy-weight shirts, thick tights, thick underwear, thick warm-up (top and pants), gloves, thick mittens, thick ski mask, hat over the ears, Vaseline covering any exposed skin, thick socks, other foot protection as needed
-20°C or °F	Add layers as needed

various outfits that make you feel better and motivate you to get into your Rx Run-Walk even on bad weather days. It is also okay to give yourself a fashionable outfit as a reward for following Rx Run-Walk regularly for several weeks.

Health Journal

The journal is such an important component in reaching health goals that we have written an entire chapter about it and provided physician-designed pages in the appendix. By using your journal to plan ahead and then later to review what you're actually doing, you are taking charge of your health! You'll find it reinforcing to write down what you did each day and will eventually miss that reinforcement if you skip.

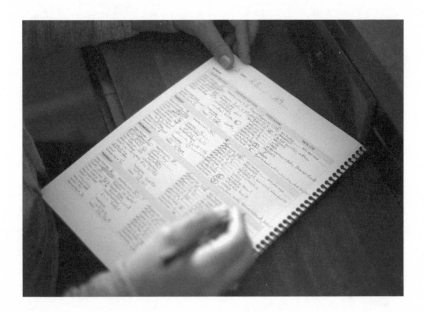

Pedometer and Watch

To obtain the information requested in the health journal, you'll need a pedometer or other device like a smart phone or watch that counts steps. You will also need a way to track time such as a stop watch.

Where to Run-Walk

The best place to start is in your neighborhood, especially if there are sidewalks. Your first priority is safety. Pick a course that is away from car traffic and is in a safe area where crime is unlikely.

Surface

By following your Rx Run-Walk training program and selecting the right shoe for you, pavement should not give extra shock to the legs or body. A smooth surface, dirt, or gravel path is a preferred surface. But beware of an uneven surface, especially if you have weak ankles or foot problems.

Picking a Run-Walk Companion

Many women who run-walk do so on their own. They enjoy the time alone. However, run-walk companions help in many ways. If you are going to run-walk with a friend at least some of the time, there are a few things to consider. Don't run-walk with someone who is faster than you unless they are fully comfortable slowing down to an easy pace that is comfortable for you. It is motivating to run with someone who will go slow enough and take a liberal amount of walking breaks so that you can talk. Share stories, jokes, or problems if you wish, and you'll bond together in a very positive way. The friendships forged on runs can be the strongest and longest lasting if you're not huffing and puffing (or puking) from trying to walk or run at a pace that is too fast for you.

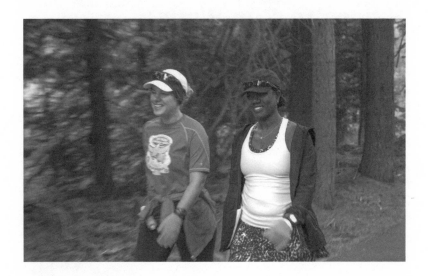

Motivation to Get Out the Door

The two most common times when walkers and runners feel challenged to follow their Rx Run-Walk are early in the morning and after work. You will find it much easier to be motivated once you experience a regular series of run-walks that make you feel good. Yes, when you run and walk at the right pace and with the right preparation, you feel better, relate to others better, and have more energy to enjoy the rest of the day.

Outside Versus Inside

Being outside is better for your overall well-being than being indoors. There are several reasons, the foremost being that the sunshine and social interaction improve your mood. However, more and more walkers and runners are using treadmills at least half of the time, particularly those who have small children. It is a fact that treadmills tend to tell you that you have gone further or faster than you really have (but they are not off by more than 10%). If you run-walk on a treadmill for the number of minutes assigned at the effort level you are used to (no huffing and puffing), you will get close enough to the training effect you wish. An elevation of 1% to 3% will help simulate a foot motion similar to running outside.

Enjoy a Cup of Joe and Maybe a Snack Before You Go

Many women using Rx Run-Walk feel better during their workouts when they have enjoyed a cup of coffee about an hour before the start. Caffeine engages the central nervous system, which gets all of the other systems needed for exercise up and running to capacity very quickly. If your blood sugar is low, which can occur in the afternoon, it might help to have a snack of about 100 to 200 calories about 30 minutes before the run-walk. Aim to make that snack be made up of 80% carbohydrates and 20% protein. Examples of such a snack include half an apple with a tablespoon of peanut butter, 8 ounces of low-fat chocolate milk, or a handful of berries with string cheese.

Care for Your Skin

We do believe the health benefits of being outside mean that we should try to exercise outside as often as the weather permits. To avoid aging your skin prematurely due to sun exposure, apply SPF 30 sunscreen at least half an hour before heading outdoors. Some women have SPF in their skin moisturizer or makeup, and that is convenient. If it's not too hot, you can also wear a wide brim hat. These forms of skin protection help reduce the risk of skin cancer.

Choose a Sports Bra

This piece of exercise equipment is just as important as shoes for comfort and exercise enjoyment for most women. A good sports bra can mean the difference been enjoying your run-walk or being absolutely miserable due to swinging breasts, bouncing, or chafing. To prevent breast pain, be prepared to pay more than you would pay for your everyday bra. There are a growing number of bras designed for specific types of exercise based upon cup size. Choose a bra specific to running. Many of the well-constructed workout bras for use during yoga, Pilates, or tennis are not supportive or comfortable for some women. The elastic in these products allows for significant bouncing and stress when walking at a brisk pace or running. Comfortable running bras tend to have microfibers that lie next to your body and move moisture away from your skin. This helps reduce chafing. For C, D, and E cups, compression bras don't work. Look for brands that have cup sizing and straps that have minimal or no elastic. Strap placement will differ among individuals, so try on a variety of bras to find what works for your body. If you feel pressure on the shoulders, where the straps press down, padded straps can help. Many large breasted women have reported success with bras that have the words *max support* on the label.

Here are some tips for bra fitting from Barb Galloway:

- Overall, the bra should fit snugly but not constrict your breathing. You want to be able to breathe naturally as the bra expands horizontally. The lower middle front of the bra should be flat across your skin—snug without pressure.

- Use the middle set of hooks when trying on the bra.

- The cup should not have wrinkles. If this is the case, try a smaller cup size. Sometimes different brands have slightly different size cups.

- If breast tissue comes out of the top of the cup or the side, try a larger size.

- The bra should not force your breasts to move in any direction, or cause them to rub together. A secure fitting cup should limit the motion.

- With the bra on, move your arms as you would do when moving the way you do during your run-walks. You shouldn't have any aggravation or restriction of arm motion.

- The width is too wide if the band rides up in the back. Try lengthening the shoulder straps.

- Under the band, front and back, you should be able to insert one finger.

- Generally, you should be able to put two fingers under each strap.

- Try it on and move the way you do during your run-walks in front of the mirror to see if there is too much bounce.

- Run-walk for at least a short distance if the store staff will let you. Ensure that you have no places that irritate, that breathing is comfortable, and that you can naturally move through the range of motion you will be doing during exercise.

- If chafing is a problem or if a hot spot develops, there are many effective blister protection products sold in convenience stores or as over-the-counter products at pharmacies.

Rules of the Road

- Shoes must be comfortable.

- No huffing or puffing.

- Don't under- or overdress.

- Talk and walk.

- Run if you feel good.

- If it hurts, slow down or take a breather.

- Keep a smile on your face and a positive attitude!

- Remember…chin up, shoulders back, and lead with your heart.

Women's Health Considerations During Run-Walk and Weight Loss

Clothing Yourself When Your Size Keeps Changing

It's thrilling when your waistline shrinks so much you discover you need the next size or two (or three) down. As some of our clients have found, it's not so thrilling when your running tights slip down on a long run and cause unexpected chaffing in the wrong places. It's also not fun to spend good money on clothes that stop fitting after just three months. If you are changing clothing sizes rapidly because you're adjusting to body changes, we recommend investing in less expensive options, borrowing from friends, or accepting hand-me-downs.

Painful Breasts

Due to changing hormones, many women find that their breasts are more sensitive at certain times of the month than others. This is because hormone changes cause the breasts to enlarge slightly. A more supportive bra may provide more comfort when this occurs.

Chafing Issues

During warm weather and on longer run-walks, most women have a few areas where clothing or body parts produce wear on other body parts. By reducing the friction in these areas, you'll reduce irritation. The most common rubbed areas are between the legs, the lower front center area of the bra, and just below and behind the shoulder where the upper arm swings behind the body. You can significantly reduce both friction and aggravation by using Vaseline and exercise products like BodyGlide that tend to last longer. Many women who have chafing problems apply lubricant to both skin surfaces and the garment before the workout, and some carry a Ziploc bag with the lubricant. As in most continuous rubbing situations, the sooner you reduce the friction, the less the irritation. Compression tights (shorts made of Lycra) reduce chafing between the legs dramatically. Sometimes too much material or seaming in the shorts or top will increase chafing. Minimal material is best.

How to Deal With Your Menstrual Cycle Whether You Have It or Not

Most women will find that regularly exercising using Rx Run-Walk helps make the issues related to a menstrual period better. Bleeding becomes more regular and less painful. Exercise can cause several different changes to a woman's period. For women who have no periods due to a condition called polycystic ovarian syndrome (PCOS), Rx Run-Walk and weight loss using Rx Eat may result in a return to regular periods. For women who exercise the way professional athletes do, periods sometimes stop.

The level of exercise and degree of calorie restriction prescribed in this book will *not* cause periods to stop, a condition called amenorrhea. The most common cause of amenorrhea in women of reproductive age is pregnancy. If your period stops while you are doing this program, see your doctor as soon as possible.

We recommend you strategically chart a route with bathrooms, bring extra tampons, and wear dark shorts or pants.

Menopause

Most women who are going through menopause find they feel better and have a better attitude on the days when they run-walk. Exercise helps women sleep better, combating insomnia and sleeping problems that are all too common during menopause.

Leaking Urine

The process of childbirth, aging, and the reduction of estrogen often results in a natural weakening of support in the lower pelvis. It is fairly common for women to experience leakage of urine, called stress urinary incontinence, during Rx Run-Walk. If one of your goals is to find your healthy weight, you should know that studies have shown that weight loss of just 8% will improve stress urinary incontinence by 50% (NEJM 2009). We also recommend all women do Kegel exercises to help strengthen pelvic muscles. Here's one guide on Kegel exercises for women: www.mayoclinic.org/healthy-lifestyle/womens-health/in-depth/kegel-exercises/art-20045283.

While weight loss and pelvic muscle strengthening take time to help urinary incontinence, don't wait to get started with Rx Run-Walk. Here are some ways women have told us they cope:

- Wear dark shorts and bring a change of clothing for use after exercise.

- Carefully reduce fluid intake for an hour or two before exercise.

- Use an absorbent pad in your shorts.

- Use the restroom right before you leave to run-walk.

Tip: If urine leaks when you laugh, cough, or increase your run-walk pace, placing a support in the vagina may help. Some women find placing a tampon before their run-walks helps. There are also over-the-counter products that can be inserted into the vagina to help provide bladder support.

Staying Safe From Motor Vehicles

Each year runners and walkers are hit by cars when exercising. Most of these are preventable. Here are the primary reasons and what you can do about them:

1. The driver is intoxicated or preoccupied by a cellphone. Always be on guard—even when walking or running on a sidewalk or pedestrian trail.

2. The runner-walker dashes across an intersection against the traffic light. When running or walking with another person, don't try to follow blindly across an intersection. When you get to an intersection, STOP. Never assume that someone ahead of you is watching out for your safety.

3. Sometimes, runner-walkers wander out into the street as they talk. Every exerciser in a group needs to be responsible for her own safety.

4. If you're in an area with cars, consider not wearing headphones or leaving one ear piece out so you can hear what's going on around you and stay tuned in to traffic.

Dog Safety

When you enter a dog's territory, you might be in for a confrontation. Here are suggestions for dealing with your dog days:

1. There are several good devices that help deter dogs: an old-fashioned stick, rocks, some electronic signal devices, and pepper spray. If you are in a new area, or an area of known dogs, Jeff recommends you have one of these at all times.

2. At the first sign of a dog ahead, try to figure out where the dog is located, whether the dog is a real threat, and what territory the dog is guarding.

3. The best option is to walk or run a different route.

4. Watch the tail. If the tail does not wag—beware.

5. As you approach the dog, it is natural for the dog to bark and head toward you. Raise your rock as if you will throw it at the dog. In Jeff's experience, the dog withdraws about 90% of the time. You may need to do this several times before getting through the dog's territory. Keep your arms up.

6. In a few cases you will need to throw the rock, and sometimes another if the dog keeps coming.

7. In less than 1% of the hundreds of dog confrontations Jeff has had, there is something wrong with the dog, and it continues to move toward you. Usually the hair will be up on the dog's back. Try to find a barrier to get behind, yell loudly in hopes the owner or someone will help you.

8. Develop your own voice. Some use a deep commanding voice, some use a high-pitched voice. Whichever you use, exude confidence and command.

Human Threats

Human threats vary widely, ranging from unwanted car horn beeps, verbal comments, and unfortunately, physical assault. Walking and running during daylight hours and in places where there are others around is helpful but does not ensure unwanted interaction. Many women have told us they have been verbally demeaned for walking and running when they are trying to lose weight. This bad behavior is inexcusable. Never let someone else's bad behavior hurt your spirit. Ignore these negative people and proceed with your workout as planned. Tell a friend what has happened to you, so you can get the emotional support you need to rejuvenate. You may be surprised that your friend is able to relate to the situation.

If there comes a day when you are physically concerned for your safety, here is some advice for self-defense.

1. Try to avoid the danger you sense by taking an alternate route or heading close to other people.

2. Use a loud, deep, commanding voice to shout, "Hey you, get away!" It really doesn't matter what you say as long as you say it loudly. Some women find having a mental rehearsal for what to do and say just in case is helpful.

3. Run-walk with a cellphone if you have one, and have 911 at the ready.

4. If you have pepper spray, use it.

5. If you have to—fight, bite, kick, and scream.

6. Have a failsafe. Always let someone else know what route you take and when you expect to return.

Bad Weather

Hot, humid days make it hard to breathe. Rainy, windy, stormy days can make exercising cold, wet, and miserable. These are days when you might consider running-walking indoors on a treadmill or water-running in a pool. If you decide to weather the weather, know that you will need to drink more fluid to keep up with sweat. You'll need more breaks—take them!

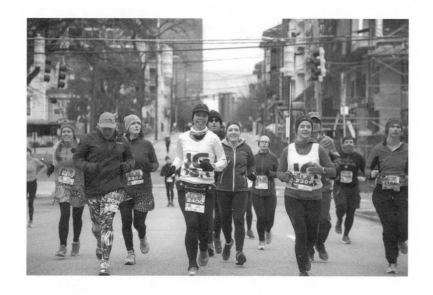

CHAPTER 3
FIND THE RX
RUN/WALK
THAT'S RIGHT
FOR YOU

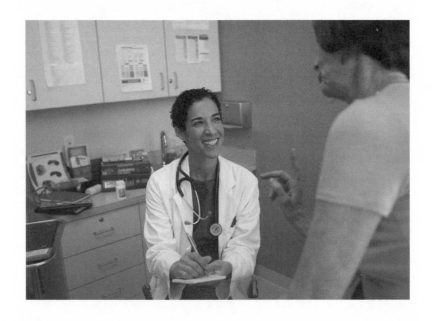

In our view, using Rx Run-Walk is just like taking medicine. Let us explain briefly why we feel confident prescribing Rx Run-Walk for you. First, Rx Run-Walk is ideally suited to achieving activity levels recommended by the United States Physical Activity Guidelines Advisory Committee (150 minutes [2.5 hours] of moderate intensity physical activity every week). Rx Run-Walk is based on guidelines and evidence, just like medicine. Next, there is a specific amount of run-walk you need to take during the week to improve many health conditions. We think of this amount of run-walk as a dose, just like there are doses for medications. Finally, if you don't take your Rx Run-Walk, it doesn't work—just like if you miss your medication, it can't help. You have to follow the instructions carefully to get the effect you want.

Running and walking consistently is enough to attain better biomarkers (health numbers) and feel better. When used consistently over 12 weeks, the gentle exercise of Rx Run-Walk changes the brain on a neurochemical basis resulting in better energy, a happier outlook, and positivity. That's why we believe the vast majority of women can improve their health using Rx Run-Walk and also why we want you to start an Rx Run-Walk training program whether or not you decide to change other parts of your life. However, you should know that when combined with adequate sleep (Rx Sleep) and healthy eating (Rx Eat), weight loss often results from Rx Run-Walk. Weight loss provides additional health and wellness. Rx Run-Walk is one kind of endurance exercise that protects against loss of muscle which means you lose weight in fat rather than muscle.

Keep Track of Your Steps— You Have to Move

Everyone needs a pedometer and should record their total number of steps every day during the 30-week program. Regardless of which prescription program you are following, aim to get at least 5,000 to 6,000 steps per day every day. More is better!

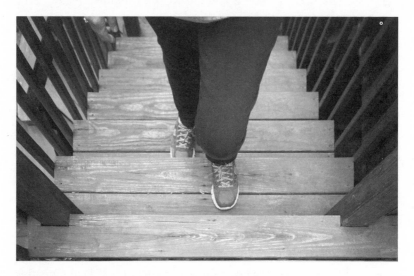

How Do I Start? Which Rx Run/Walk Is Right for Me?

Because we start at different points, we need to find what fits your baseline health now so you can start a training program that fits with where you are. Over the next 30 weeks, the right training program will help you gradually reach the full dose of Rx Run-Walk. So let's find which of the three Rx Run-Walk programs is best for you—Rx Get Started, Rx Keep Going, or Rx Burn Fat. Answer a couple screening questions, then use the chart below to see which chapters are most relevant to your health needs.

R$_X$ Run/Walk — BURN FAT

Ruth Parker, MD and Carmen Mohan, MD
Better Health
Atlanta, GA 30307

Name: _____ Age: _____
Address: _____
Date: _____

R$_X$ Take a Run/Walk at a pace of about 20 min per mile
in ideal weather according to the schedule below:

M	Tu	Wed	Th	F	Sat	Sun
REST	60 min (3 miles)	REST	60 min (3 miles)	60 min (3 miles)	REST	100 min (5 miles)

Indications:

- ☑ Restore bones, joints, and muscles
- ☑ Improve mood, mental well-being, coping
- ☑ Get more restorative sleep
- ☑ Improve heart health and circulation
- ☑ Improve thinking and remembering
- ☑ Breathe more easily
- ☑ Improve cholesterol
- ☑ Control blood sugar
- ☑ Lower blood pressure
- ☑ Find my healthy weight

Signature *Ruth M. Parker, MD*   *Carmen Patrick Mohan, MD*

R$_X$ Run/Walk — KEEP GOING

Ruth Parker, MD and Carmen Mohan, MD
Better Health
Atlanta, GA 30307

Name: _____ Age: _____
Address: _____
Date: _____

R$_X$ Take a Run/Walk at a pace of about 20 min per mile
in ideal weather according to the schedule below:

M	Tu	Wed	Th	F	Sat	Sun
REST	30 min (1.5 miles)	REST	30 min (1.5 miles)	30 min (1.5 miles)	REST	60 min (3 miles)

Indications:

- ☑ Restore bones, joints, and muscles
- ☐ Improve mood, mental well-being, coping
- ☐ Get more restorative sleep
- ☑ Improve heart health and circulation
- ☑ Improve thinking and remembering
- ☑ Breathe more easily
- ☑ Improve cholesterol
- ☑ Control blood sugar
- ☑ Lower blood pressure
- ☐ Find my healthy weight

Signature *Ruth M. Parker, MD*   *Carmen Patrick Mohan, MD*

R$_X$ Run/Walk — GET STARTED

Ruth Parker, MD and Carmen Mohan, MD
Better Health
Atlanta, GA 30307

Name: _____ Age: _____
Address: _____
Date: _____

R$_X$ Take a 30-minute Walk 5 times a week with as many
breaks as you need for a total of 2.5 miles a week
in ideal weather according to the schedule below:

M	Tu	Wed	Th	F	Sat	Sun
30 min (0.5 miles)	30 min (0.5 miles)	REST	30 min (0.5 miles)	30 min (0.5 miles)	30 min (0.5 miles)	REST

Indications:

- ☑ Restore bones, joints, and muscles
- ☐ Improve mood, mental well-being, coping
- ☐ Get more restorative sleep
- ☑ Improve heart health and circulation
- ☐ Improve thinking and remembering
- ☑ Breathe more easily
- ☐ Improve cholesterol
- ☐ Control blood sugar
- ☐ Lower blood pressure
- ☐ Find my healthy weight

Signature *Ruth M. Parker, MD*   *Carmen Patrick Mohan, MD*

Find the HER Prescription that is Right for You

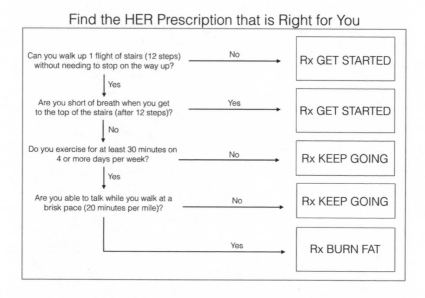

The prescriptions reflect the level of Rx Run-Walk you will be able to master by the end of the matching Rx Run-Walk training program. Each course feeds into the next course. For example, if you were routed into Keep Going it means you are likely ready to begin Week 1 of the Keep Going training program. After 30 weeks of consistently using the Keep Going training program, you will reach the full dose of Rx Run-Walk needed to create fundamental health.

One word of caution. We haven't met any woman who doesn't want to burn fat. The trouble is that burning fat through Rx Run-Walk requires a certain level of fitness and time. If you try to ignore where you really are, and start in a program that isn't right for you, you'll end up injured. Don't do this. Instead, realize that you'll be able to do the Burn Fat program in time. After about 12 to 16 weeks of taking Rx Run-Walk at full dose, you should consider coming back to the Find Your Prescription Tool. It's likely you'll be ready to begin the next training program, Burn Fat.

Training Program for the Rx Run/Walk—Get Started

Steps for Getting Started

This program assumes you partner with your doctor as you do the program.

1. Talk to your doctor.

2. Show your doctor the training schedule.

3. Ask your doctor if any modifications are recommended.

4. Be sure you understand and know how to follow instructions for all of your medications.

5. Do NOT begin this program if you require supplemental oxygen from a home oxygen tank OR you have been hospitalized in the last month.

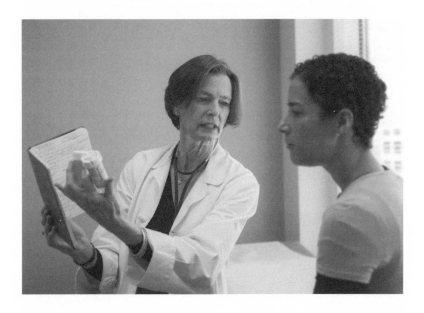

What to Expect

By the end of this 30-week Rx Run-Walk: Get Started training program, you will have laid the foundation for improving mobility and increasing your body's ability to metabolize energy.

Training Program Outline and Structure

The first four weeks of the Get Started training program are a quick start to cultivating an exercise habit. Beneath the number of the week, you will see the total walking time allotted for the week. The program begins with week 1 in which you will walk for 40 minutes total. The program ends with week 30 in which you will walk for 150 minutes total, thereby reaching the full dose of prescribed exercise.

Remaining injury-free is the single most important predictor of improvement in walking endurance. To succeed in this program, you must embrace the following principle: the body builds itself *after* a challenge while it is at rest. This means you should take breaks as many times as you need and for as long as you need to catch your breath. We can't emphasize this principle enough. If you take a break BEFORE you feel fatigued, you will not only help to build your ability to walk for a longer time, but you will also prevent injury.

In this program, every minute you spend walking counts toward your daily time. If you park your car at the grocery store and walk inside, that minute counts toward your daily goal. By the end of your walks, you should feel like you could go for at least 2 more minutes if needed. You should NOT feel completely exhausted. Maintain a pace that is right for you so that you are feeling good at the end of each day. Remember: NO huffing and puffing.

What Are Recovery Weeks?

You may notice that every fifth week is a lower duration week. This is intentional. These weeks will help your body build muscle and strengthen tendons—two of the most injury-prone parts of the body. For this reason, we call lower duration weeks *recovery weeks*. Weeks 5, 10, 15, 20, and 25 are recovery weeks. During recovery weeks, focus on obtaining the recommended 7 or more hours of sleep nightly, maintaining good nutrition, taking good care of any weak links, and treating any aches appropriately.

What Are Maintenance Weeks?

The last four weeks are *maintenance weeks*. They are there so you can prove to yourself that maintaining your prescribed run-walk schedule is not only well within your grasp, but you've been able to handle it well for almost a month!

You have a great deal of control over the part of life that revolves around exercise if you choose to take charge. The way you schedule your walks, your rewards, and your challenges will significantly influence your motivation. You can also control how good you feel during each walk and how quickly you recover.

Motivation Tips

✓ Find a place in your schedule when you are very likely to have time to walk. For most people this means getting up 40 minutes earlier. Don't skimp on sleep! Instead, go to bed 40 minutes earlier. Even better, go to sleep an hour earlier. Your body needs the restorative sleep anyway.

✓ Get your spouse, significant other, friends, co-workers, etc., to be your support team. Promise that if you get through the next three weeks having done the run-walks, you will have a party for them, or a picnic, or whatever! Pick supportive people who will email you, and will be supportive during and after the training, and during the celebration.

✓ Have a friend or three who you can call in case you have a low motivation day. Just the voice on the phone can usually get you out the door. Of course, it is always best to have a positive and enthusiastic person in this role.

✓ It is best to also have a backup time to walk. The usual back-up times are at noon or after work.

✓ Break your walk into several segments if necessary.

There is no need to ever experience pain in a walking program. But this puts on you, the new walker, the responsibility of a slow enough pace and frequent enough rests. You can have fun when you walk—every single time—if you don't spend all of the resources early. That said, we do make recommendations for duration of the walking segments you attempt. The recommended duration of walking before taking a break gradually increases every five weeks. If you are finding you consistently need a break before the recommended walk segment is up, your body probably needs more time to adapt to your new exercise program. Count back four weeks in the training schedule, and try those weeks again. You may need to do this a number of times, or once early on as you get started and again mid-schedule like in weeks 18 or 24.

What to Do During the Rest Break

Plan scheduled breaks but remember you can always take another break if you need it. Scheduled breaks should be 1 to 3 minutes each (longer if needed). Some days, you'll need more rest, some days you'll need less. This is part of learning your body and its needs. During the break, you can walk at a much slower pace—essentially just shuffling your feet low to the ground—sit down, or just stand still long enough to feel recovered. Raise your arms over your head. Prepare your mind by saying this mantra aloud or silently to yourself, "Lead with your heart. Smile on your face. Wind at your back." Focus on your breathing. Build energy for the next walk segment.

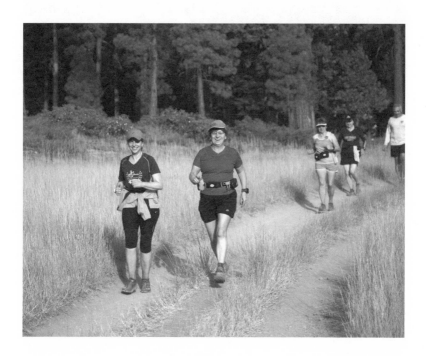

Your First Week: How to Begin and Continue

The most important week is your first week, and it only takes 30 seconds to get started!

The truth is any amount of activity is better than sitting around. Standing up is better for you than sitting. Walking is better than standing. Even if you walk for just 30 seconds before sitting back down, it's better for your health than doing nothing at all.

It's time to learn by doing. Here is a first-time-out instruction list that will ease you into walking—a shakedown cruise for your body.

A Caffeine Boost?

To get the mind ready for exercise, many walkers have a cup of coffee, tea, or diet drink about an hour before they walk. If your blood sugar level is low due to any reason (especially in the afternoon), eat about half of an energy bar or drink 100-200 calories of a sports drink—especially one that has about 20% protein—about 25-30 minutes before the start of the run. If you have problems with caffeine, don't use it.

The First Walk on Monday

1. Put on a pair of comfortable walking shoes.

2. Put on light comfortable clothes. Note: Clothes don't have to be designed for exercise—just comfortable.

3. Set a timer for 30 seconds. The timer can be your watch, phone, or an egg timer, or you can just count 30 steps.

4. Walk for 30 seconds at a slow enough pace to keep your breathing easy. You should be able to talk as you walk.

5. Take a break. Stand still and rest. Sit down if you need to. Take as long as you need to catch your breath, cool down, and feel comfortable again.

6. Alternate 30 seconds of walking at a comfortable pace with the breaks you need.

7. Do this for a total of 8 minutes walking—no more.

8. Use a gentle stride, which is relaxed and not long.

For example, you might start with a 30-second walk and need 2 minutes of rest followed by a walk of 30 seconds, then another minute of rest. Next, walk 30 seconds followed by 2 minutes of rest, walk 30 seconds then another minute of rest. The total time spent walking would be 2 minutes. Those 2 minutes would count toward your goal of 8 minutes of walking. You might then decide to take an extended break and come back during your lunch hour for a workout with a different pattern—walk 30 seconds, rest 30 seconds, walk 30 seconds, rest 30 seconds—alternating in this fashion for a total of 12 repeats which would give you another 6 minutes of walking time. That's it— you've reached your goal of 8 minutes total walking time for the day.

Again, only you can decide how much rest you need to keep your breathing even and easy. Maybe you need only 10 to 15 seconds of rest, maybe you need several minutes to catch your breath. You will make considerable gains by sticking to your walking time goals no matter how long your break times are.

The Second Walk on Tuesday

Repeat the same routine as the first time but reduce the total walk time to 6 minutes.

Wednesday

Rest completely. Let your body recover.

The Third Walk on Thursday

You're back to the routine again. Repeat the alternating 30 second walk-break cycle you did on your first walk for a total time of 8 minutes spent walking.

The Fourth Walk on Friday

You're in the groove now—just 6 minutes total to do today, 30 seconds at a time.

The Fifth Walk on Saturday

This is the challenge day. You're going to walk for 12 minutes total. Do this in any fashion you can, with walks no more than 30 seconds at a time. For example, if you feel too fatigued after 6 minutes of walk-rest, go ahead and take a long break—even if it means several hours go by before you try again. It's the cumulative (total) time spent walking that matters. Just make sure you get to the total time of 12 minutes.

Reward Yourself!

After you have finished your first week, congratulate yourself with a special walking outfit, meal, or trip to a great walking area or park. Remember that rewards can be very powerful.

Congratulations! You're on your way to becoming a regular walker!

Your Three-Week Schedule

If there is any time in your life when you adjust your schedule so that you can exercise, this is it!

If you can maintain the next three weeks of walking (only 15 days of walking), you have about an 80% chance of continuing walking for 6 months. And if you make it to the six-month club, you will tend to continue as a life-long walker.

Here are some tips for your 21-day mission:

- Schedule your run-walk days at least two weeks in advance.

- Commit to the prescribed schedule of Tuesdays, Thursdays, Fridays, and Sundays. Get out there on the designated days. If you wait until the spirit moves you to walk, you will probably have many empty spaces in your training journal.

- Pick a time when the temperature is okay for you and a time period you usually have open. Lock it in!

- Plan. You must also be in charge of the little things that keep the schedule filled, such as spending a few minutes each week to plan your weekly walks and to reward yourself afterward.

- Journal! The commitment to yourself to simply get out there four times a week will be reinforced significantly by writing it down.

- Stick to it! Regularity is important for the body and the mind. When you have three exercise-free days between walks, you start to lose some of your walking conditioning and adaptations.

Week 2

Mission: You are continuing to increase distance. On Saturday, pick a scenic place for your workout. Each day, repeat the 30-second walk and 1- to 3-minute rest cycle to reach the total walking time goal listed below:

Monday: 8 minutes

Tuesday: 6 minutes

Thursday: 8 minutes

Friday: 6 minutes

Saturday: 16 minutes

Week 3

Mission: You're really making progress now! On Saturday, ask some friends to go with you for the walk and have a picnic afterward. You've made it 3 weeks! Keep going, you have an easy week coming. Each day, repeat the 30-second walk and 1- to 3-minute rest cycle to reach the total walking time goal listed below:

Monday: 10 minutes

Tuesday: 6 minutes

Thursday: 8 minutes

Friday: 8 minutes

Saturday: 18 minutes

Week 4

Mission: It's time for your 3-week party. Pick the day and the place, and celebrate the fact you're able to walk 20 minutes! Each day, repeat the 30-second walk and 1- to 3-minute rest cycle to reach the total walking time goal listed below:

Monday: 10 minutes

Tuesday: 6 minutes

Thursday: 8 minutes

Friday: 6 minutes

Saturday: 20 minutes

Week 5

Mission: Time for your first recovery week. Rest a bit. You've earned it! Plus, your body needs it to prepare for the next part of your journey.

Monday: 8 minutes

Tuesday: 6 minutes

Thursday: 8 minutes

Friday: 6 minutes

Saturday: 12 minutes

Where to Go From Here?

It's time to increase the duration of the walk segments and gradually remove the breaks. Starting with week 6, the recommended duration of the walk segment increases every 5 weeks. However, you should determine the amount of walking-resting each day that allows you to feel good with no aches and pains. Shoot for goals that are within your reach but also challenging. Remember, no huffing and puffing! Add more walking and less resting but keep the huffing under control.

If you have not yet been able to walk for 30 seconds continuously, don't worry. This means your body needs more time to adjust. To reduce the chance of injury, start the training program again beginning with week 1. You should also talk with your doctor about this training program, show your doctor your journal pages, and ask for further recommendations to keep you on the Rx Run-Walk path.

Congratulations on completing your Rx Run-Walk: Get Started training program! You are walking enough to

- ✓ restore bones, joints, and muscles;
- ✓ breathe more easily; and
- ✓ improve heart health and circulation.

You can continue to enhance these health benefits by consistently following your walking prescription for 12 weeks.

After 12 weeks of following the Rx Run-Walk: Get Started training program, it's time to make plans to continue. The Keep Going training program starts to increase the distance you cover by gradually removing the breaks you're allowed to take. We invite you to consider starting the Keep Going training program when you feel good for at least 12 weeks (i.e., one season) of taking the prescribed Get Started walks at full dose (week 30). When you're thinking about moving on to the training program for the Keep Going course, take a moment to revisit chapter 3 to see if the Keep Going course is right for you.

Fill this out and post it on the fridge!

R$_X$ Run/Walk — GET STARTED

Ruth Parker, MD and Carmen Mohan, MD
Better Health
Atlanta, GA 30307

Name: _____   Age: _____
Address: _____
Date: _____

R$_X$ Take a 30-minute Walk 5 times a week with as many breaks as you need for a total of 2.5 miles a week in ideal weather according to the schedule below:

M	Tu	Wed	Th	F	Sat	Sun
30 min (0.5 miles)	30 min (0.5 miles)	REST	30 min (0.5 miles)	30 min (0.5 miles)	30 min (0.5 miles)	REST

Indications:

☑ Restore bones, joints, and muscles   ☑ Breathe more easily

☐ Improve mood, mental well-being, coping   ☐ Improve cholesterol

☐ Get more restorative sleep   ☐ Control blood sugar

☑ Improve heart health and circulation   ☐ Lower blood pressure

☐ Improve thinking and remembering   ☐ Find my healthy weight

Signature *Ruth M. Parker, MD*   *Carmen Patrick Mohan, MD*

Training Schedule for Rx Run-Walk: Get Started*

Week #	Mon	Tues	Wed	Thurs	Fri	Sat	Sun
Week 1	Walk for 8 minutes in 30-second segments	Walk for 6 minutes in 30-second segments	OFF	Walk for 8 minutes in 30-second segments	Walk for 6 minutes in 30-second segments	Walk for 12 minutes in 30-second segments	OFF
Week 2	Walk for 8 minutes in 30-second segments	Walk for 6 minutes in 30-second segments	OFF	Walk for 8 minutes in 30-second segments	Walk for 6 minutes in 30-second segments	Walk for 16 minutes in 30-second segments	OFF
Week 3	Walk for 10 minutes in 30-second segments	Walk for 6 minutes in 30-second segments	OFF	Walk for 8 minutes in 30-second segments	Walk for 6 minutes in 30-second segments	Walk for 18 minutes in 30-second segments	OFF
Week 4	Walk for 10 minutes in 30-second segments	Walk for 6 minutes in 30-second segments	OFF	Walk for 8 minutes in 30-second segments	Walk for 8 minutes in 30-second segments	Walk for 20 minutes in 30-second segments	OFF
Week 5	Walk for 8 minutes in 30-second segments	Walk for 6 minutes in 30-second segments	OFF	Walk for 8 minutes in 60-second segments	Walk for 6 minutes in 30-second segments	Walk for 12 minutes in 30-second segments	OFF
Week 6	Walk for 10 minutes in 60-second segments	Walk for 8 minutes in 60-second segments	OFF	Walk for 10 minutes in 60-second segments	Walk for 8 minutes in 60-second segments	Walk for 20 minutes in 60-second segments	OFF

	Day 1	Day 2	Day 3	Day 4	Day 5	Day 6	Day 7
Week 7	Walk for 12 minutes in 60-second segments	Walk for 8 minutes in 60-second segments	OFF	Walk for 10 minutes in 60-second segments	Walk for 8 minutes in 60-second segments	Walk for 24 minutes in 60-second segments	OFF
Week 8	Walk for 12 minutes in 60-second segments	Walk for 10 minutes in 60-second segments	OFF	Walk for 12 min in 60-second segments	Walk for 10 minutes in 60-second segments	Walk for 24 minutes in 60-second segments	OFF
Week 9	Walk for 14 minutes in 90-second segments	Walk for 10 minutes in 90-second segments	OFF	Walk for 14 minutes in 90-second segments	Walk for 10 minutes in 90-second segments	Walk for 26 minutes in 90-second segments	OFF
Week 10	Walk for 6 minutes in 90-second segments	Walk for 10 minutes in 90-second segments	OFF	Walk for 6 minutes in 90-second segments	Walk for 10 minutes in 90-second segments	Walk for 15 minutes in 90-second segments	OFF
Week 11	Walk for 15 minutes in 2-minute segments	Walk for 12 minutes in 2-minute segments	OFF	Walk for 15 minutes in 2-minute segments	Walk for 10 minutes in 2-minute segments	Walk for 26 minutes in 2-minute segments	OFF
Week 12	Walk for 15 minutes in 2-minute segments	Walk for 15 minutes in 2-minute segments	OFF	Walk for 15 minutes in 2-minute segments	Walk for 12 minutes in 2-minute segments	Walk for 28 minutes in 2-minute segments	OFF

Week #	Mon	Tues	Wed	Thurs	Fri	Sat	Sun
Week 13	Walk for 15 minutes in 2-minute segments	Walk for 15 minutes in 2-minute segments	OFF	Walk for 15 minutes in 2-minute segments	Walk for 15 minutes in 2-minute segments	Walk for 30 minutes for 2-minute segments	OFF
Week 14	Walk for 15 minutes in 2-minute segments	Walk for 20 minutes in 2-minute segments	OFF	Walk for 15 minutes in 2-minute segments	Walk for 20 minutes in 2-minute segments	Walk for 30 minutes in 2-minute segments	OFF
Week 15	Walk for 10 minutes in 2-minute segments	Walk for 10 minutes in 2-minute segments	OFF	Walk for 10 minutes in 2-minute segments	Walk for 10 minutes in 2-minute segments	Walk for 25 minutes in 2-minute segments	OFF
Week 16	Walk for 15 minutes in 3-minute segments	Walk for 12 minutes in 3-minute segments	OFF	Walk for 15 minutes in 3-minute segments	Walk for 12 minutes in 3-minute segments	Walk for 30 minutes in 3-minute segments	OFF
Week 17	Walk for 20 minutes in 3-minute segments	Walk for 15 minutes in 3-minute segments	OFF	Walk for 20 minutes in 3-minute segments	Walk for 15 minutes in 3-minute segments	Walk for 30 minutes in 3-minute segments	OFF
Week 18	Walk for 20 minutes in 3-minute segments	Walk for 20 minutes in 3-minute segments	OFF	Walk for 20 minutes in 3-minute segments	Walk for 20 minutes in 3-minute segments	Walk for 30 minutes in 3-minute segments	OFF

Week 19	Walk for 25 minutes in 3-minute segments	Walk for 20 minutes in 3-minute segments	OFF	Walk for 25 minutes in 3-minute segments	Walk for 20 minutes in 3-minute segments	Walk for 30 minutes in 3-minute segments	OFF
Week 20	Walk for 10 minutes in 3-minute segments	Walk for 15 minutes in 3-minute segments	OFF	Walk for 15 minutes in 3-minute segments	Walk for 10 minutes in 3-minute segments	Walk for 20 minutes in 3-minute segments	OFF
Week 21	Walk for 20 minutes in 4-minute segments	Walk for 15 minutes in 4-minute segments	OFF	Walk for 20 minutes in 4-minute segments	Walk for 15 minutes in 4-minute segments	Walk for 30 minutes in 4-minute segments	OFF
Week 22	Walk for 25 minutes in 4-minute segments	Walk for 20 minutes in 4-minute segments	OFF	Walk for 25 minutes in 4-minute segments	Walk for 20 minutes in 4-minute segments	Walk for 30 minutes in 4-minute segments	OFF
Week 23	Walk for 25 minutes in 4-minute segments	Walk for 25 minutes in 4-minute segments	OFF	Walk for 25 minutes in 4-minute segments	Walk for 25 minutes in 4-minute segments	Walk for 30 minutes in 4-minute segments	OFF
Week 24	Walk for 30 minutes in 4-minute segments	Walk for 25 minutes in 4-minute segments	OFF	Walk for 30 minutes in 4-minute segments	Walk for 25 minutes in 4-minute segments	Walk for 30 minutes in 4-minute segments	OFF

Week #	Mon	Tues	Wed	Thurs	Fri	Sat	Sun
Week 25	Walk for 15 minutes in 4-minute segments	Walk for 15 minutes in 4-minute segments	OFF	Walk for 15 minutes in 4-minute segments	Walk for 15 minutes in 4-minute segments	Walk for 25 minutes in 4-minute segments	OFF
Week 26	Walk for 25 minutes in 5-minute segments	Walk for 20 minutes in 5-minute segments	OFF	Walk for 25 minutes in 5-minute segments	Walk for 20 minutes in 5-minute segments	Walk for 30 minutes in 5-minute segments	OFF
Week 27	Walk for 30 minutes in 5-minute segments	Walk for 25 minutes in 5-minute segments	OFF	Walk for 30 minutes in 5-minute segments	Walk for 25 minutes in 5-minute segments	Walk for 30 minutes in 5-minute segments	OFF
Week 28	Walk for 30 minutes in 5-minute segments	Walk for 30 minutes in 5-minute segments	OFF	Walk for 30 minutes in 5-minute segments	Walk for 30 minutes in 5-minute segments	Walk for 30 minutes in 5-minute segments	OFF
Week 29	Walk for 30 minutes in 5-minute segments	Walk for 30 minutes in 5-minute segments	OFF	Walk for 30 minutes in 5-minute segments	Walk for 30 minutes in 5-minute segments	Walk for 30 minutes in 5-minute segments	OFF
Week 30	Walk for 30 minutes (0.5 miles)	Walk for 30 minutes (0.5 miles)	OFF	Walk for 30 minutes (0.5 miles)	Walk for 30 minutes (0.5 miles)	Walk for 30 minutes (0.5 miles)	OFF

*Post this on your fridge!

Training Program for Rx Run/Walk—Keep Going

Before you embark on this training program, you should be able to walk at a conversational pace for at least 5 minutes without needing a break.

1. Look at week 1. If the long walk for Sunday on week 1 exceeds your current ability, we recommend you begin with the training program for the Get Started course.

2. Show your doctor the training schedule.

3. Ask your doctor if any modifications would be recommended.

4. Be sure you understand and know how to follow instructions for all of your medications.

What to Expect

By the end of this 30-week Rx Run-Walk: Keep Going training program, you will be able to run-walk at the level required to maintain the fundamentals of health.

Training Program Outline and Structure

The first eight weeks of Rx Run-Walk: Keep Going build the foundation for walking endurance. While we recommend specific durations for both the walking segments and the break segments, you should take breaks before you feel fatigued to help increase your ability to walk longer distances. The program begins with week 1 in which you will walk for 40 minutes total. The program ends with week 30 in which you will walk for 150 minutes total thereby reaching the full dose of prescribed exercise. By the end of your walks, you should feel like you would be able to walk for at least 5 to 10 more minutes if needed.

That is, you should NOT feel completely exhausted. Maintain a pace that is right for you so that you are feeling good at the end of each workout.

Remaining injury-free is the single most important predictor of improvement in walking endurance. To succeed in this program, you must embrace the following principle: the body builds itself *after* a challenge while it is at rest.

We can't emphasize breaks enough. If you take a break BEFORE you feel fatigued, you will not only cultivate your ability to walk for a longer time, but you will also prevent injury. There is no need to ever experience pain in a walking program. But this puts on you, the new walker, the responsibility of a slow enough pace and frequent enough rests. You can have fun when you walk—every single time—if you don't spend all of your resources early.on as you get started and again mid-schedule like in weeks 18 or 24.

That said, we do make recommendations for the number of breaks you take to stop and rest or even sit down if you need to. The recommended duration of walking before taking a break gradually increases every five weeks. If you are finding you consistently need more breaks than the training schedule recommends, your body probably needs more time to adapt to your new exercise program. Count back four weeks in the training schedule, and try those weeks again. You may need to do this a number of times, or once early on as you get started and again mid-schedule like in weeks 18 or 24.

During this program, you are asked to run on some of the Sunday walks. By run, we mean pick up your pace from a comfortable walk at conversational pace to a brisk walk where you can still talk albeit in short sentences. Remember: NO huffing and puffing. You can also consider a jog (or shuffle) for the recommended run segments.

Note: The shuffle is a motion between running and walking. From a walk, you would shorten your stride, keep your feet low to the ground and pick up the cadence. The ankle should do most of the work so that the muscles don't have to do much work.

During weeks 25 through 29, you'll notice the increased time and frequency of the run segments. These weeks will help you increase your speed and gradually build up to the recommended 20-minute mile pace.

What Are Recovery Weeks?

You will notice this plan will gradually increase week to week and then suddenly go down on the total run-walk time. This is intentional. These lower duration weeks will help your body build muscle and strengthen tendons. For this reason, we call them *recovery weeks*. Weeks 7, 11, 16, 22, and 26 are recovery weeks. During these weeks, focus on obtaining the recommended 7 or more hours of sleep nightly, maintaining good nutrition, taking good care of any weak links, and treating any aches appropriately.

What Are Maintenance Weeks?

The last four weeks are *maintenance weeks*. They are there so you can prove to yourself that maintaining your prescribed run-walk schedule is not only well within your grasp, but you've been able to handle it well for over a month!

Motivation Tips

✓ Find a place in your schedule when you are very likely to have time to walk. For most people this means getting up 40 minutes earlier. Don't skimp on sleep! Instead, go to bed 40 minutes earlier. Even better, go to sleep an hour earlier. Your body needs the restorative sleep anyway.

✓ Get your spouse, significant other, friends, co-workers, etc., to be your support team. Promise that if you get through the next 3 weeks having done the run-walks, you will have a party for them, or a picnic, or whatever! Pick supportive people who will email you, and will be supportive during and after the training, and during the celebration.

✓ Have a friend or three who you can call in case you have a low motivation day. Just the voice on the phone can usually get you out the door. Of course, it is always best to have a positive and enthusiastic person in this role.

✓ It is best to also have a backup time to walk. The usual back-up times are at noon or after work.

✓ Break your walk into several segments if necessary.

Tips on Form as You Run-Walk

When you walk, one foot is on the ground at any time. Running in any form means that there will be a second or less when both feet are off the ground. This requires a bit more effort. Most beginners can insert a few short jogs of 5-10 seconds, after a few weeks of walking. But if you aren't comfortable doing this, just alternate between a gentle walk and a brisk walk.

Note on stride length: Whether walking or jogging, don't use a long stride. Keep the feet low to the ground, touch lightly and keep the stride fairly short (see the folowing photos). This allows the ankle to do a lot of the work, reducing stress on the muscles, joints, and feet.

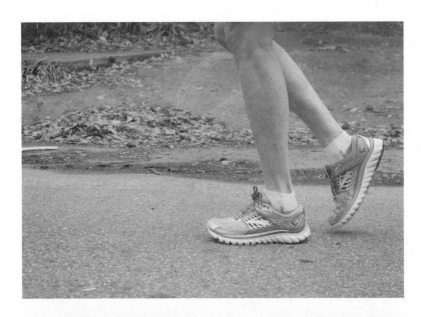

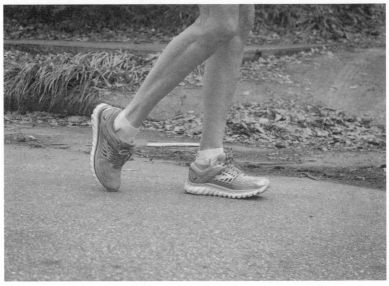

What to Do During the Walk Break

The training program recommends scheduled breaks, but remember that you can always take another break if you need it. Scheduled breaks should be 1 to 3 minutes each (longer if needed). Some days, you'll need more rest, some days you'll need less. This is part of learning your body and its needs. During the break, you can walk at a much slower pace—essentially just shuffling your feet low to the ground. You can also sit down, or stand still long enough to feel recovered. Raise your arms over your head. Prepare your mind by saying this mantra aloud or silently to yourself, "Lead with your heart. Smile on your face. Wind at your back." Focus on your breathing. Build energy for the next walk segment.

Your First Week: How to Begin and Continue

The most important week is your first week, and it only takes 12 minutes to get started!

It's time to learn by doing. Here is a first run-walk instruction list that will ease you into the program—a shakedown cruise for your body.

A Caffeine Boost?

To get the mind ready for exercise, many walkers have a cup of coffee, tea, or diet drink about an hour before they walk. If your blood sugar level is low due to any reason (especially in the afternoon), eat about half of an energy bar or drink 100-200 calories of a sports drink—especially one that has about 20% protein—about 25-30 minutes before the start of the run. If you have problems with caffeine, don't use it.

Monday

Prepare your mind for your new schedule. Make a list of reasons you want to become a regular walker. Think of some of your challenges and make a plan for how to manage them so you achieve the daily goals. This will be useful in maintaining your motivation in the coming days.

The First Walk on Tuesday

1. Put on a pair of comfortable walking shoes.

2. Put on light comfortable clothes. Note: Clothes don't have to be designed for exercise—just comfortable.

3. Set a timer for 5 minutes. The timer can be on your watch or phone.

4. Walk for 5 minutes at a slow enough pace to keep your breathing easy. You should be able to talk as you walk.

5. Take a break. Stand still and rest. Sit down if you need to. The recommended break duration is 2 minutes, but take as long as you need to catch your breath, cool down, and feel comfortable again.

6. Do it again. Walk for 5 minutes at your own pace.

7. You're done! You've walked for 10 minutes total.

Wednesday

Rest completely. Let your body recover.

The Second Walk on Thursday

Repeat the same routine as the first time but reduce the total walk time to 5 minutes.

The Third Walk on Friday

You're back to the routine again. Repeat the alternating 5-minute walk and 2-minute break cycle you did on your first walk for a total time of 10 minutes spent walking.

Saturday

Another day off for complete rest.

The Fourth Walk on Sunday

You're in the groove now! Walk for 5 minutes, take a break for 2 minutes (longer if needed), and repeat the walk-break cycle 3 times for a total of 15 minutes spent walking.

Reward Yourself!

After you have finished your first week, congratulate yourself with a special walking outfit, meal, or trip to a great walking area or park. Remember that rewards can be very powerful.

Congratulations! You're on your way to becoming a regular walker!

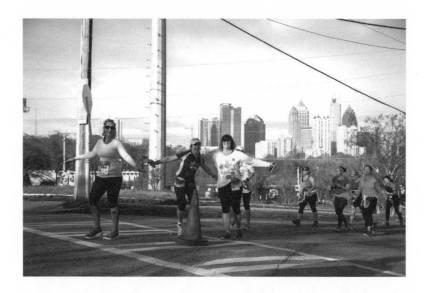

Your Three-Week Schedule

If there is any time in your life when you adjust your schedule so that you can exercise, this is it!

If you can maintain the next three weeks of walking (only 12 days of walking), you have about an 80% chance of continuing walking for 6 months. And if you make it to the six-month club, you will tend to continue as a life-long walker.

Here are some tips for your 21-day mission:

- Schedule your run-walk days at least two weeks in advance.

- Commit to the prescribed schedule of Tuesdays, Thursdays, Fridays, and Sundays. Get out there on the designated days. If you wait until the spirit moves you to walk, you will probably have many empty spaces in your training journal.

- Pick a time when the temperature is okay for you and a time period you usually have open. Lock it in!

- Plan. You must also be in charge of the little things that keep the schedule filled, such as spending a few minutes each week to plan your weekly walks and to reward yourself afterward.

- Journal! The commitment to yourself to simply get out there four times a week will be reinforced significantly by writing it down.

- Stick to it! Regularity is important for the body and the mind. When you have three exercise-free days between walks, you start to lose some of your walking conditioning and adaptations.

Week 2

Mission: You are continuing to increase distance. On Sunday, pick a scenic place for your workout. Each day, alternate the 5-minute walk with a break of 2 minutes to reach the total walking time goal listed below:

Tuesday: 10 minutes

Thursday: 5 minutes

Friday: 10 minutes

Sunday: 20 minutes

Week 3

Mission: You're really making progress now! On Sunday, ask some friends to go with you for the walk and have a picnic afterward. You've made it 3 weeks. Keep going! On the weekdays, alternate the recommended walk segment with a break of 2 minutes to reach the total walking time goal listed here:

Tuesday: 15 minutes

Thursday: 5 minutes

Friday: 10 minutes

Sunday: 10 minutes (Note: Breaks are removed and runs are introduced on this workout. You are up to the challenge!)

Week 4

Mission: It's time for your 3-week party. Pick the day and the place, and celebrate the fact that you're able to walk 25 minutes! On the weekdays, alternate the recommended walk segment with a break of 2 minutes to reach the total walking time goal listed below:

Tuesday: 15 minutes

Thursday: 10 minutes

Friday: 10 minutes

Sunday: 25 minutes (Note: This is the challenge day which improves your endurance. Take as many breaks as you need for as long as you need to reach the total walking time.)

Week 5

Mission: Time for your first recovery week. Rest a bit. You've earned it.

Tuesday: 5 minutes

Thursday: 10 minutes

Friday: 15 minutes

Sunday: Alternate walking 3 minutes with a run of 30 seconds for a total time of 10 minutes and 30 seconds

NOTE: The gentlest running form is a shuffle. Keep your feet low to the ground with a light touch and a short stride. This will give you a slight increase in exertion without overwhelming the feet, legs, and joints.

Where to Go From Here? Gradually Removing Breaks

It's time to increase the duration of the walk segments and gradually remove the breaks. Starting with week 6, the recommended duration of the walk segment increases every 2 weeks. However, you should determine the amount of walking and resting each day that allows you to feel good with no aches and pains. Shoot for goals that are within your reach but also challenging. Remember, no huffing and puffing! Add more walking and less resting but keep the huffing under control.

Note: There is no goal in this program to keep increasing the running every workout. While the short run segments improve mental activity and fitness, if you are challenged by a given amount of running, take a 5-minute walk and start over with shorter run segments.

If you have not yet been able to walk continuously for 10 minutes, don't worry. This means your body needs more time to adjust. To reduce the chance of injury, start the training program again beginning with week 1. You should also talk with your doctor about this training program, show your doctor your journal pages, and ask for further recommendations to keep you on the Rx Run-Walk path.

Training Schedule for Rx Run-Walk: Keep Going

Week #	Mon	Tues	Wed	Thurs	Fri	Sat	Sun
Week 1	OFF	Walk for 5 minutes Break for 2 minutes Walk for 5 minutes	OFF	Walk for 5 minutes	Walk for 5 minutes Break for 2 minutes Walk for 5 minutes	OFF	Repeat 3 times (Walk for 5 minutes Break for 2 minutes)
Week 2	OFF	Walk for 5 minutes Break for 2 minutes Walk for 5 minutes	OFF	Walk for 5 minutes	Walk for 5 minutes Break for 2 minutes Walk for 5 minutes	OFF	Repeat 4 times (Walk for 5 minutes Break for 2 minutes)
Week 3	OFF	Walk for 7 minutes Break for 2 minutes Walk for 8 minutes	OFF	Walk for 5 minutes	Walk for 5 minutes Break for 2 minutes Walk for 5 minutes	OFF	Repeat 2 times (Walk for 5 minutes Run for 30 seconds)
Week 4	OFF	Walk for 7 minutes Break for 2 minutes Walk for 8 minutes	OFF	Walk for 5 minutes Break for 2 minutes Walk for 5 minutes	Walk for 5 minutes Break for 2 minutes Walk for 5 minutes	OFF	25-minute walk with as many breaks as needed

Week #	Mon	Tues	Wed	Thurs	Fri	Sat	Sun
Week 5	OFF	Walk for 5 minutes	OFF	Walk for 10 minutes	Repeat 3 times (Walk for 5 minutes Break for 2 minutes)	OFF	Repeat 3 times (Walk for 3 minutes Run for 30 seconds)
Week 6	OFF	Walk for 7 minutes Break for 2 minutes Walk for 8 minutes	OFF	Walk for 10 minutes	Walk for 7 minutes Break for 2 minutes Walk for 8 minutes	OFF	Walk for 10 minutes Break for 2 minutes Walk for 10 minutes Break for 2 minutes Walk for 10 minutes
Week 7	OFF	Walk for 5 minutes	OFF	Walk for 15 minutes with as many breaks as needed	Walk for 7 minutes Break for 1 minute Walk for 8 minutes	OFF	Repeat 3 times (Walk for 5 minutes Run for 30 seconds)
Week 8	OFF	Repeat 4 times (Walk for 5 minutes Break for 1 minute)	OFF	Walk for 7 minutes Break for 1 minute Walk for 8 minutes	Walk for 7 minutes Break for 1 minute Walk for 8 minutes	OFF	Walk for 35 minutes with as many breaks as needed

Week 9	OFF	Walk for 5 minutes	OFF	Walk for 15 minutes	Walk for 8 minutes Break for 1 minute Walk for 8 minutes Break for 1 minute Walk for 4 minutes	OFF	Walk for 7 minutes Run for 1 minute Walk for 8 minutes Run for 1 minute
Week 10	OFF	Walk for 8 minutes Break for 1 minute Walk for 8 minutes Break for 1 minute Walk for 4 minutes	OFF	Walk for 8 minutes Break for 1 minute Walk for 8 minutes Break for 1 minute Walk for 4 minutes	Walk for 8 minutes Break for 1 minute Walk for 8 minutes Break for 1 minute Walk for 4 minutes	OFF	Walk for 40 minutes with as many breaks as needed
Week 11	OFF	Walk for 5 minutes	OFF	Walk for 20 minutes with as many breaks as needed	Walk for 8 minutes Break for 1 minute Walk for 8 minutes Break for 1 minute Walk for 4 minutes	OFF	Repeat 3 times (Walk for 5 minutes Run for 1 minute)

Week #	Mon	Tues	Wed	Thurs	Fri	Sat	Sun
Week 12	OFF	Walk for 10 minutes Break for 1 minute Walk for 10 minutes Break for 1 minute Walk for 5 minutes	OFF	Walk for 10 minutes Break for 1 minute Walk for 10 minutes	Walk for 10 minutes Break for 1 minute Walk for 10 minutes	OFF	Walk for 45 minutes with as many breaks as needed
Week 13	OFF	Walk for 5 minutes	OFF	Walk for 10 minutes Break for 1 minute Walk for 15 minutes	Walk for 10 minutes Break for 1 minute Walk for 15 minutes	OFF	Repeat 4 times (Walk for 5 minutes Run for 1 minute)
Week 14	OFF	Walk for 25 minutes	OFF	Walk for 25 minutes	Walk for 25 minutes	OFF	Walk for 20 minutes
Week 15	OFF	Walk for 10 minutes Break for 1 minute Walk for 15 minutes Break for 1 minute Walk for 5 minutes	OFF	Walk for 25 minutes	Walk for 25 minutes	OFF	Walk for 50 minutes with as many breaks as needed
Week 16	OFF	Repeat 2 times (Walk for 5 minutes Run for 30 seconds)	OFF	Walk for 25 minutes	Walk for 20 minutes	OFF	Repeat 4 times (Walk for 5 minutes Run for 1 minute)

	Day 1	Day 2	Day 3	Day 4	Day 5	Day 6	Day 7
Week 17	OFF	Walk for 15 minutes Break for 1 minute Walk for 15 minutes	OFF	Walk for 15 minutes Break for 1 minute Walk for 15 minutes	Walk for 15 minutes Break for 1 minute Walk for 15 minutes	OFF	Walk for 15 minutes Break for 1 minute Walk for 15 minutes
Week 18	OFF	Walk for 30 minutes	OFF	Walk for 30 minutes	Walk for 20 minutes	OFF	Walk for 55 minutes with as many breaks as needed
Week 19	OFF	Walk for 10 minutes	OFF	Walk for 30 minutes	Walk for 20 minutes	OFF	Repeat 5 times (Walk for 5 minutes Run for 1 minute)
Week 20	OFF	Walk for 10 minutes Run for 30 seconds Walk for 10 minutes Run for 30 seconds Walk for 10 minutes	OFF	Walk for 30 minutes	Walk for 30 minutes	OFF	Walk for 30 minutes
Week 21	OFF	Walk for 10 minutes Run for 30 seconds Walk for 10 minutes Run for 30 seconds Walk for 10 minutes	OFF	Walk for 30 minutes	Walk for 20 minutes	OFF	Repeat 4 times (Walk for 15 minutes Break for 2 minutes)

Week #	Mon	Tues	Wed	Thurs	Fri	Sat	Sun
Week 22	OFF	Walk for 10 minutes	OFF	Walk for 30 minutes	Walk for 25 minutes	OFF	Walk for 35 minutes
Week 23	OFF	Repeat 4 times (Walk for 7 minutes Run for 30 seconds Walk for 2 minutes)	OFF	Walk for 30 minutes	Walk for 20 minutes	OFF	Repeat 6 times (Walk for 4 minutes Run for 1 minute)
Week 24	OFF	Walk for 30 minutes	OFF	Walk for 30 minutes	Walk for 30 minutes	OFF	Walk for 15 minutes Break for 1 minute Walk for 15 minutes Break for 1 minute Walk for 10 minutes
Week 25	OFF	Repeat 4 times (Walk for 6 minutes Run for 1 minute) Walk for 2 minutes	OFF	Walk for 30 minutes	Repeat 4 times (Walk for 6 minutes Run for 1 minute) Walk for 2 minutes	OFF	Repeat 3 times (Walk for 15 minutes Break for 1 minute) Walk for 15 minutes

Week 26	OFF	Walk for 30 minutes	OFF	Walk for 30 minutes	OFF	Walk for 30 minutes	OFF	Walk for 30 minutes
Week 27	OFF	Repeat 6 times (Walk for 4 minutes Run for 1 minute)	OFF	Walk for 30 minutes	OFF	Repeat 6 times (Walk for 4 minutes Run for 1 minute)	OFF	Repeat 3 times (Walk for 7 minutes Run for 2 minutes) Walk for 3 minutes
Week 28	OFF	Walk for 30 minutes	OFF	Walk for 30 minutes	OFF	Walk for 30 minutes	OFF	Walk for 15 minutes Break for 1 to 3 minutes Walk for 30 minutes Break for 1 to 3 minutes Walk 15 minutes
Week 29	OFF	Repeat 3 times (Walk for 8 minutes Run for 2 minutes)	OFF	Walk for 30 minutes	OFF	Repeat 6 times (Walk for 4 minutes Run for 1 minute)	OFF	Walk for 30 minutes
Week 30	OFF	Walk for 30 minutes (1.5 miles)	OFF	Walk for 30 minutes (1.5 miles)	OFF	Walk for 30 minutes (1.5 miles)	OFF	Walk for 60 minutes (3 miles)

Post this on your fridge!

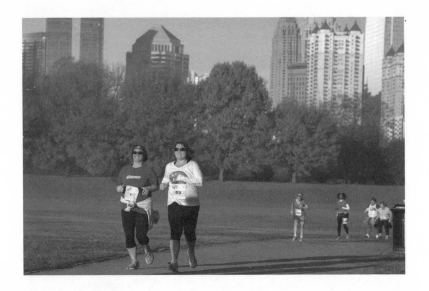

Congratulations on completing your Keep Going training program! You are walking enough to

✓ restore bones, joints, and muscles;

✓ improve heart health and circulation;

✓ improve thinking and remembering;

✓ breathe more easily;

✓ improve cholesterol;

✓ control blood sugar; and

✓ lower blood pressure.

Good news! You can further enhance these health benefits by consistently following your walking prescription.

Fill this out and post it on your fridge!

R_x Run/Walk — KEEP GOING

Ruth Parker, MD and Carmen Mohan, MD
Better Health
Atlanta, GA 30307

Name: _____ Age: _____
Address: _____
Date: _____

R_x Take a Run/Walk at a pace of about 20 min per mile
in ideal weather according to the schedule below:

M	Tu	Wed	Th	F	Sat	Sun
REST	30 min (1.5 miles)	REST	30 min (1.5 miles)	30 min (1.5 miles)	REST	60 min (3 miles)

Indications:

- [✓] Restore bones, joints, and muscles
- [ ] Improve mood, mental well-being, coping
- [ ] Get more restorative sleep
- [✓] Improve heart health and circulation
- [✓] Improve thinking and remembering

- [✓] Breathe more easily
- [✓] Improve cholesterol
- [✓] Control blood sugar
- [✓] Lower blood pressure
- [ ] Find my healthy weight

Signature *Ruth M. Parker, MD*   *Carmen Patrick Mohan, MD*

Now it's time to make plans on how to keep going even further. Continue the week 30 prescription dose for 12 weeks. This will give you the level of fitness required to start the Fat Burning training program. The Fat Burning training program gradually increases the amount of time you are able to run-walk so you perform the level of exercise required to burn off excess fat and begin to develop a leaner physique.

We invite you to consider starting the Fat Burning training program when you feel good for at least 12 weeks (i.e., one season) of taking the run-walks prescribed in week 30 of the Keep Going training program. When you're thinking about moving on to the Fat Burning training program, take a moment to revisit chapter 3 to see if you meet the other prerequisites.

Get bonus points! Go be a spectator at a 5K or 10K near you. Watch what happens at the finish line. Think "that could be me." You can find a race online or through Jeff's website: www.jeffgalloway.com The Barb 5K is a particular favorite of ours.

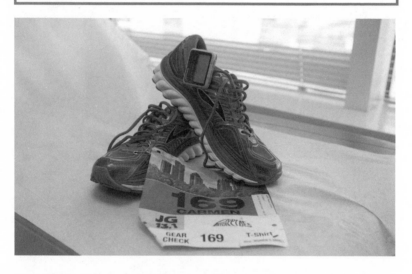

Training Program for Rx Run/Walk—Burn Fat

Steps for Getting Started

Before you embark on this training program, you should be able to walk at a conversational pace (about 20 minutes per mile) for at least 60 minutes with only a short break if you take one at all.

1. Look at week 1. If the long walk for Sunday on week 1 exceeds your current ability, we recommend you begin with the Keep Going training program.

2. Show your doctor the training schedule.

3. Ask your doctor if any modifications are recommended.

4. Be sure you understand and know how to follow instructions for all of your medications.

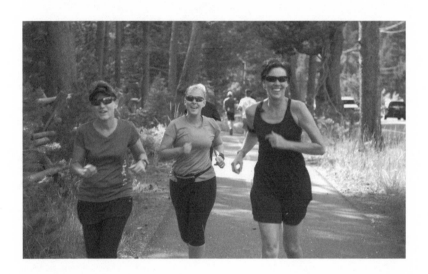

What to Expect

By the end of this 30-week course, you will be able to use run-walk to gain recreational fitness. In addition, you will lose about 0.5 to 1 pound of fat weekly because you are also following the Rx Eat: Burn Fat.

Course Outline and Structure

The first eight weeks of the Fat Burning training program expand the foundation for walking endurance from 60 minutes to 90 minutes.

This amount of walking is required because fat is metabolized only after the first 30 to 45 minutes of walking. One 90-minute walk will burn anywhere between 300 and 450kcal of fat. To lose one pound, a woman needs to burn about 500kcal per day, or about 3500 kcal weekly.

The program begins with week 1 in which you will walk for 150 minutes total. The program ends with week 30 in which you will run-walk for 280 minutes total, thereby reaching the full dose of prescribed exercise. By the end of your run-walk, you should feel like you would be able to walk for at least 5 to 10 more minutes if needed. That is, you should NOT feel completely exhausted. Maintain a pace that is right for you so that you are feeling good at the end of each workout.

This program gradually builds your walking endurance over 20 weeks before introducing run segments in week 21. By *run*, we mean pick up your pace from a comfortable walk at conversational pace to a brisk walk where you can still talk albeit in short sentences. Remember: NO huffing and puffing. You can also consider a jog for the recommended run segments or consider the shuffle.

Note: The shuffle is a motion between running and walking. From a walk, you would shorten your stride, keep your feet low to the ground and pick up the cadence. The ankle should do most of the work so that the muscles don't have to do much work.

By week 28, you should adjust the ratio of walking time versus running time. A certain number of run segments are recommended, but you get to decide how long you want them to be. A total run-walk time is recommended.

Motivation Tips

- ✓ Find a place in your schedule when you are very likely to have time to walk. For most people this means getting up 40 minutes earlier. Don't skimp on sleep! Instead, go to bed 40 minutes earlier. Even better, go to sleep an hour earlier. Your body needs the restorative sleep anyway.

- ✓ Get your spouse, significant other, friends, co-workers, etc., to be your support team. Promise that if you get through the next 3 weeks having done the run-walks, you will have a party for them, or a picnic, or whatever! Pick supportive people who will email you, and who will be supportive during and after the training, and during the celebration.

- ✓ Have a friend or three who you can call in case you have a low motivation day. Just the voice on the phone can usually get you out the door. Of course, it is always better to have a positive and enthusiastic person in this role.

- ✓ It is best to also have a backup time to walk. The usual backup times are at noon or after work.

- ✓ Break your walk into several segments if necessary.

Tips on Form as You Run-Walk:

When you walk, one foot is on the ground at any time. Running in any form means that there will be a second or less when both feet are off the ground. This requires a bit more effort. Most beginners can insert a few short jogs of 5-10 seconds, after a few weeks of walking. But if you aren't comfortable doing this, just alternate between a gentle walk and a brisk walk.

Note on stride length: Whether walking or jogging, don't use a long stride. Keep the feet low to the ground, touch lightly and keep the stride fairly short. This allows the ankle to do a lot of the work, reducing stress on the muscles, joints, and feet.

Your First Week: How to Begin and Continue

The most important week is your first week, it only takes 30 minutes to get started!

It's time to learn by doing. Here is a first run-walk instruction list that will ease you into the program—a shakedown cruise for your body.

A Caffeine Boost?

To get the mind ready for exercise, many walkers have a cup of coffee, tea, or diet drink about an hour before they walk. If your blood sugar level is low due to any reason (especially in the afternoon), eat about half of an energy bar or drink 100-200 calories of a sports drink—especially one that has about 20% protein—about 25-30 minutes before the start of the run. If you have problems with caffeine, don't use it.

Monday

Prepare your mind for your new schedule. Make a list of reasons you want to become a regular run-walker. Think of some of your challenges and make a plan for how to manage them so you achieve the daily goals. This will be useful in maintaining your motivation in the coming days.

The First Walk on Tuesday

1. Put on a pair of comfortable walking shoes.

2. Put on light comfortable clothes. Note: Clothes don't have to be designed for exercise—just comfortable.

3. Set a timer for 30 minutes. The timer can be on your watch or phone.

4. Walk for 30 minutes at a slow enough pace to keep your breathing easy. You should be able to talk as you walk.

Wednesday

Rest completely. Let your body recover.

The Second Walk on Thursday

Repeat the same routine as the first time.

The Third Walk on Friday

You're back to the routine again; walk 30 minutes.

Saturday

Another day off for complete rest.

The Fourth Walk on Sunday

You're in the groove now! Walk for 60 minutes, ideally in a scenic place you enjoy.

Reward Yourself!

After you have finished your first week, congratulate yourself with a special walking outfit, meal, or trip to a great walking area or park. Remember that rewards can be very powerful.

Congratulations! You're on your way to fat burning!

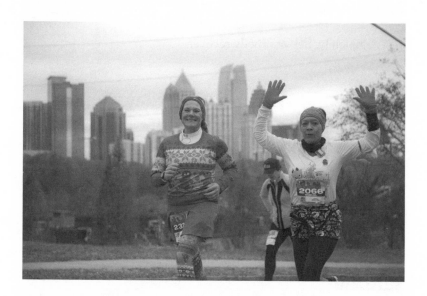

Your Three-Week Schedule

If there is any time in your life when you adjust your schedule so that you can exercise, this is it!

If you can maintain the next three weeks of walking (only 12 days of walking), you have about an 80% chance of continuing walking for 6 months. And if you make it to the six-month club you will tend to continue as a life-long walker. Here are some tips for your 21-day mission:

- Schedule your run-walk days at least two weeks in advance

- Commit to the prescribed schedule of Tuesdays, Thursdays, Fridays, and Sundays. Get out there on the designated days. If you wait until the spirit moves you to walk, you will probably have many empty spaces in your training journal.

- Pick a time when the temperature is okay for you and a time period you usually have open. Lock it in!

- Plan. You must also be in charge of the little things that keep the schedule filled, such as spending a few minutes a week to plan your weekly walks and to reward yourself afterward.

- Journal! The commitment to yourself to simply get out there four times a week will be reinforced significantly by writing it down.

- Stick to it! Regularity is important for the body and the mind. When you have three exercise-free days between walks, you start to lose some of your walking conditioning and adaptations.

Week 2

Mission: You are ready to increase distance. On Sunday, pick a scenic place for your workout.

For each day, walk for the total time goal listed below:

Tuesday: 35 minutes

Thursday: 30 minutes

Friday: 40 minutes

Sunday: 60 minutes

Week 3

Mission: You're really making progress now! On Sunday, ask some friends to go with you for the walk and have a picnic afterward. You've made it 3 weeks. Keep going!

Tuesday: 40 minutes

Thursday: 35 minutes

Friday: 40 minutes

Sunday: 65 minutes

Week 4

Mission: It's time for your 3-week party. Pick the day and the place, and celebrate the fact you're able to walk 70 minutes!

Tuesday: 45 minutes

Thursday: 35 minutes

Friday: 40 minutes

Sunday: 70 minutes (This is the challenge day which improves your endurance. Take as many breaks as you need for as long as you need to reach the total walking time.)

Week 5

Mission: Time for your first recovery week. Rest a bit. You've earned it.

Tuesday: 35 minutes

Thursday: 30 minutes

Friday: 40 minutes

Sunday: 60 minutes

Where to Go From Here? Increasing the Pace and Gradually Introducing Runs

Time to further increase the duration of the walk segments and gradually quicken your pace so you can start to run. You should determine the amount of walking and running each day that allows you to feel good with no aches and pains. Shoot for goals that are within your reach but that are also challenging. Remember, no huffing and puffing! Add slower walking or shuffling when needed to keep the huffing under control.

If you have not yet been able to walk continuously for 70 minutes, don't worry. This means your body needs more time to adjust. To reduce the chance of injury, start the training program again beginning with week 1. You should also talk with your doctor about this training program, show your doctor your journal pages, and ask for further recommendations to keep you on the walking path.

Congratulations on completing your Burn Fat training program! You are now run-walking enough to

- ✓ restore bones, joints, and muscles;
- ✓ improve mood, mental well-being, and coping;
- ✓ get more restorative sleep;
- ✓ improve heart health and circulation;
- ✓ improve thinking and remembering;
- ✓ breathe more easily;
- ✓ improve cholesterol;

✓ control blood sugar;

✓ lower blood pressure; and

✓ find your healthy weight.

Good news! You can further enhance these health benefits by consistently following your Rx Run-Walk prescription.

Fill this out and post it on your fridge!

R_X Run/Walk — BURN FAT

Ruth Parker, MD and Carmen Mohan, MD
Better Health
Atlanta, GA 30307

Name: _____   Age: _____
Address: _____
Date: _____

R_X Take a Run/Walk at a pace of about 20 min per mile in ideal weather according to the schedule below:

M	Tu	Wed	Th	F	Sat	Sun
REST	60 min (3 miles)	REST	60 min (3 miles)	60 min (3 miles)	REST	100 min (5 miles)

Indications:

☑ Restore bones, joints, and muscles   ☑ Breathe more easily

☑ Improve mood, mental well-being, coping   ☑ Improve cholesterol

☑ Get more restorative sleep   ☑ Control blood sugar

☑ Improve heart health and circulation   ☑ Lower blood pressure

☑ Improve thinking and remembering   ☑ Find my healthy weight

Signature *Ruth M. Parker, MD*   *Carmen Patrick Mohan, MD*

Now it's time to make plans on how to keep going. Decide on your weight loss goal. Continue the week 30 prescription dose for the number of weeks equal to the number of pounds you want to lose. It's likely you still have miles to go and you'll want some company. Research shows that women who exercise with a group are more likely to stick with their programs. You are now ready to join a Jeff Galloway training group or related program. Visit www.JeffGalloway. com and click on "Training Programs" for more information.

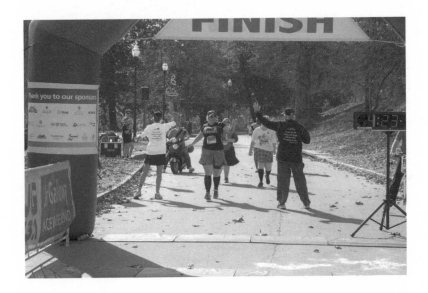

Training Schedule for Rx Run-Walk: Burn Fat*

Week #	Mon	Tues	Wed	Thurs	Fri	Sat	Sun
Week1	OFF	30 minutes (1.5 miles)	OFF	30 minutes (1.5 miles)	30 minutes (1.5 miles)	OFF	60 minutes (3 miles)
Week 2	OFF	35 minutes	OFF	30 minutes	40 minutes	OFF	60 minutes
Week 3	OFF	40 minutes	OFF	35 minutes	40 minutes	OFF	65 minutes
Week 4	OFF	45 minutes	OFF	35 minutes	40 minutes	OFF	70 minutes
Week 5	OFF	35 minutes	OFF	30 minutes	40 minutes	OFF	60 minutes
Week 6	OFF	45 minutes	OFF	35 minutes	40 minutes	OFF	70 minutes
Week 7	OFF	45 minutes	OFF	45 minutes	45 minutes	OFF	70 minutes
Week 8	OFF	50 minutes	OFF	50 minutes	50 minutes	OFF	80 minutes
Week 9	OFF	50 minutes	OFF	50 minutes	60 minutes	OFF	90 minutes
Week 10	OFF	40 minutes	OFF	35 minutes	40 minutes	OFF	65 minutes
Week 11	OFF	45 minutes	OFF	45 minutes	45 minutes	OFF	75 minutes
Week 12	OFF	50 minutes	OFF	50 minutes	50 minutes	OFF	80 minutes
Week 13	OFF	50 minutes	OFF	55 minutes	65 minutes	OFF	95 minutes
Week 14	OFF	60 minutes	OFF	55 minutes	65 minutes	OFF	95 minutes
Week 15	OFF	45 minutes	OFF	45 minutes	40 minutes	OFF	70 minutes
Week 16	OFF	50 minutes	OFF	50 minutes	50 minutes	OFF	80 minutes
Week 17	OFF	50 minutes	OFF	50 minutes	50 minutes	OFF	90 minutes
Week 18	OFF	60 minutes	OFF	60 minutes	50 minutes	OFF	90 minutes

Week 19	OFF	60 minutes	OFF	60 minutes	OFF	60 minutes	OFF	100 minutes
Week 20	OFF	50 minutes	OFF	45 minutes	OFF	45 minutes	OFF	80 minutes
Week 21	OFF	Repeat 5 times (Walk for 8 minutes Run for 1 minute) Walk for 5 minutes	OFF	Repeat 5 times (Walk for 8 minutes Run for 1 minute) Walk for 5 minutes	OFF	Repeat 5 times (Walk for 8 minutes Run for 1 minute) Walk for 5 minutes	OFF	Walk for 15 minutes Repeat 5 times (Walk for 8 minutes Run for 1 minute) Walk for 25 minutes
Week 22	OFF	Repeat 6 times (Walk for 9 minutes Run for 1 minute)	OFF	Repeat 6 times (Walk for 9 minutes Run for 1 minute)	OFF	Repeat 5 times (Walk for 9 minutes Run for 1 minute)	OFF	Walk for 15 minutes Repeat 5 times (Walk for 9 minutes Run for 1 minute) Walk for 25 minutes
Week 23	OFF	Repeat 6 times (Walk for 9 minutes Run for 1 minute)	OFF	Repeat 6 times (Walk for 9 minutes Run for 1 minute)	OFF	Repeat 6 times (Walk for 9 minutes Run for 1 minute)	OFF	Walk for 20 minutes Repeat 5 times (Walk for 9 minutes Run for 1 minute) Walk for 20 minutes

Week #	Mon	Tues	Wed	Thurs	Fri	Sat	Sun
Week 24	OFF	Repeat 7 times (Walk for 9 minutes Run for 1 minute)	OFF	Repeat 6 times (Walk for 9 minutes Run for 1 minute)	Repeat 7 times (Walk for 9 minutes Run for 1 minute)	OFF	Walk for 20 minutes Repeat 5 times (Walk for 9 minutes Run for 1 minute) Walk for 20 minutes
Week 25	OFF	50 minutes	OFF	50 minutes	50 minutes	OFF	90 minutes
Week 26	OFF	Repeat 5 times (Walk for 8 minutes Run for 2 minutes)	OFF	Repeat 5 times (Walk for 8 minutes Run for 2 minutes)	Repeat 5 times (Walk for 8 minutes Run for 2 minutes)	OFF	Walk for 20 minutes Repeat 5 times (Walk for 9 minutes Run for 1 minute) Walk for 20 minutes
Week 27	OFF	60 minutes	OFF	55 minutes	60 minutes	OFF	95 minutes
Week 28	OFF	70 minutes with 7 or more run segments	OFF	60 minutes with 6 or more run segments	60 minutes with 6 or more run segments	OFF	100 minutes with 5 or more run segments
Week 29	OFF	60 minutes with 6 or more run segments	OFF	60 minutes with 6 or more run segments	60 minutes with 6 or more run segments	OFF	100 minutes with 5 or more run segments
Week 30	OFF	60 minutes (3 miles)	OFF	60 minutes (3 miles)	60 minutes (3 miles)	OFF	100 minutes (5 miles)

*Post this on your fridge!

CHAPTER 4
YOU GOTTA EAT—FIND YOUR RX EAT

Our Food Philosophy

Food we eat should nourish our bodies and make us feel full of the energy we need to enjoy life. Food is central to healthy living. The best things to eat for health promotion are low in sugar, not processed, and mostly made at home. Food should be eaten in as close to its natural state as possible.

Why We Like the Mediterranean Diet

Science is clear that the Mediterranean diet is associated with healthy aging and longer lifespans. The Mediterranean diet prevents diabetes. In people with diabetes, a Mediterranean diet helps control blood sugars. People who eat a Mediterranean diet are less likely to have a heart attack or stroke. They are also less likely to develop Alzheimer's disease or dementia, or be diagnosed with cancer (including breast cancer).

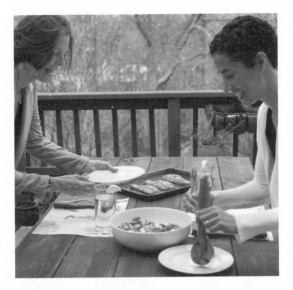

The Mediterranean diet includes the following food categories in order of most important to least important to good health:

- ✓ Fresh or frozen vegetables

- ✓ Fresh or frozen fruits

- ✓ Whole grains

- ✓ Beans

- ✓ Nuts

- ✓ Seeds

- ✓ Fish

- ✓ Poultry (turkey, chicken)

- ✓ Dairy products (full fat)

- ✓ Olive oil and healthy fats

- ✓ Honey

- ✓ *Optional*: Low to moderate amounts of wine (preferably red wine)

The following items are NOT included in a Mediterranean diet because they are bad for your health:

✗ Sugary sweets like cookies, candy, cake, pie, and ice cream

✗ Processed foods (i.e., food that comes in packages)

✗ Food you can get as take out like at fast food restaurants

✗ Soda (not even diet soda)

✗ Store-bought fruit juice

✗ Canned fruit

✗ Beer

✗ Liquor

✗ Fried food

✗ Ready-made salad dressings

✗ Red meat including beef, pork, and game like venison, buffalo, or rabbit

The following items are NOT included in a Mediterranean diet but ARE included in this weight loss program:

• Coffee

• Tea

• Dark chocolate

Food Score

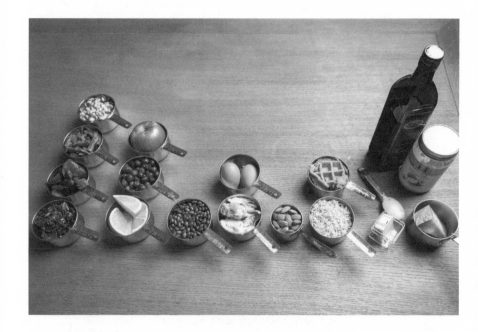

What Is Your Diet Quality and Why Does It Matter?

Diet quality is important to ensure you eat all of the nutrients needed to be healthy.

Quality foods contribute to health whether or not you lose weight. We categorize high-quality food to help you optimize the health benefits you get from food you eat. Maybe you've tasted all of these foods. Maybe some of them are unfamiliar. Eating a wide variety of food and being willing to try new foods will help you on your path to finding the highest quality foods you like, can regularly prepare on your own, and share with family and friends.

Examples of High-Quality Food by Category

Food category	Examples
Vegetables	Beets, Brussels sprouts, cabbage, carrots, cauliflower, cucumbers, garlic, ginger, lettuce, mushrooms, onions, parsnips, peas, peppers, pumpkin, squash, sweet potatoes, tomatoes, turmeric, turnips, yams, zucchini
Leafy green vegetables	Arugula (also called rocket), beet greens, bok choy, broccoli, carrot greens, collard greens, kale, mizuna, mustard greens, spinach, Swiss chard, turnip greens
Fruits	Apples, avocado, bananas, berries, dates, figs, grapes, melons, oranges, peaches, pears, pineapples, raisins
Nuts	Almonds (including almond milk), cashews, chia seeds, flax seeds, hazelnuts (including hazelnut milk), macadamia nuts, peanuts, pecans, pine nuts, pumpkin seeds, walnuts
Beans	Black beans, calypso, garbanzo beans (also called chickpeas), hummus, kidney beans, lentils, navy beans, pinto beans, soy milk, tempeh, tofu
Whole grains	Brown rice, bulgur, couscous, forbidden rice, millet, oatmeal, quinoa, wheat bread, wild rice, wheat pasta
Dairy	Cheese, plain yogurt (preferably Greek yogurt), cow or goat milk
Lean protein	Chicken, duck, eggs, fish, protein powder, turkey
Good fats	Olive oil, butter (not margarine), nut and seed oils such as coconut oil, sesame oil, peanut oil, grapeseed oil, canola oil

What Is the Food Score and How Do I Figure Mine Out?

The food score helps you judge how well you adhered to a Mediterranean diet each day. Learn how to calculate your food score below and log it in your journal every day.

The highest food score possible in one day is 8 points. You earn one point when you eat high-quality food in these amounts:

- At least 4 cups of vegetables (must include at least one leafy green and no more than 1 cup of potatoes or corn)

- At least 3 cups of fresh fruit (no more than one glass of fresh-squeezed fruit juice; one serving of dried fruit is 0.5 cups)

- 1 to 2 cups of beans

- 1 to 2 cups of lean protein

- 0.5 cups of nuts or seeds

- 2 cups of whole grains

- Up to 3 table-spoons of good fats (preferably less)

- 1 cup of dairy

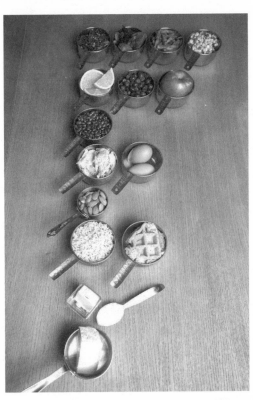

The following are cost-neutral foods (i.e., there is no change in quality points if eaten at or below recommended amounts):

- Black coffee (1 teaspoon honey okay, no other sweetener)

- Tea (1 teaspoon honey okay, no other sweetener)

- Sauces (soy sauce, sriracha sauce, ketchup, mustard)

- Vinaigrettes (balsamic, apple cider vinegar, lemon juice, olive oil, salt, pepper and spices)

- 1 glass of wine, preferably red wine

- 0.25 ounces dark chocolate (about 10 dark chocolate chips)

You lose a quality point for eating (or drinking) any of the following (e.g., if you ate one deduction from each category in one day, you would lose 8 quality points):

- Unhealthy grains such as white bread or white rice. This includes each sugary treat eaten. So eating three cookies gives you -3 points.

- Added sugar such as sugar added to tea, cereal, or other foods; sugar in the form of jelly, fruit preserves, or maple syrup; sugar substitutes like stevia or agave

- Processed foods (i.e., food that comes in packages)

- Food you can get as take out like at fast food restaurants

- Soda (including diet soda)

- Store-bought fruit juice

- Beer (12 ounces), each glass after the first glass of wine (5 ounces), or a cocktail or liquor (1.5 ounces)

- Chocolate other than dark chocolate such as milk chocolate or white chocolate, or more than 0.25 ounces of dark chocolate

Diet Quality Rules

Rule 1: Use a measuring cup. Be sure you are eating the right serving size.

Rule 2: For each of the food categories, you receive +1 point when you reach the recommended number of servings.

Rule 3: You have to eat a lot of vegetables. This one is usually the hardest point to score. It's also the most important one to score!

- To get the veggie points, you have to eat the recommended number of servings or you get no points. In fact, you get no points if you eat less than the recommended number of servings of fruits and vegetables. It's a make-it or break-it point system with no room for extra credit. For example, if you eat 4 cups of vegetables over the course of the day, you receive 1 point as long as at least one of those vegetables was a leafy green AND not more than 1 of those cups was from potato or corn.

- If you eat 5 or 6 cups of vegetables, (which we encourage you to do because it's even better for your health), it still earns you the same point. On the other hand, if you eat 3 cups of vegetables that day, you receive no points. If you eat 4 cups of vegetables but none were green OR more than 1 was a potato, you get no points.

- When you eat 1 cup of leafy green veggies, circle the tally mark to make the veggie point qualifier easier to see when you calculate your food score at the end of the day.

Rule 4: There are categories of food like nuts and dairy where you are not allowed more than a certain serving size. This is because these foods are needed in a healthy, balanced diet, but only in lower amounts. If you do not eat these foods, you are missing out on some of the nutrients you need. If you eat more of these foods than recommended, you will fall short of your weight loss goals. This is why you receive a deduction (-1 point) if you eat more than the recommended amount.

How to Determine Your Food Score for the Day

- Step 1: Keep your journal with you at all times. Give yourself a tally mark for everything you eat based on its food category.

- Step 2: If you earned a deduction (-1 point), remember to mark those down as well.

- Step 3: At the end of the day, when you have no plans to eat or drink anything more, give yourself a check when you met or exceeded the goal for a given food category.

- Step 4: Add up the number of checks. This is equal to the total positive (+) quality points for the day.

- Step 5: Add up the number of (-) deductions you got.

- Step 6: Subtract the total deductions from the total of positive quality points. You've arrived at your food score.

Let's look at a couple examples now. Compare the meal plans in the following tables to see how just a few bad food choices dramatically change your food score.

What I Ate	How to Tally		How to Score
Breakfast: 2 pieces of wheat toast with cottage cheese and 1 cup of sliced strawberries		Veggies: Fruits: I Beans: Protein: Nuts: Grains: I Good fats: Dairy: I	Veggies (4): IIII = +1 Fruits (3): III = +1 Beans (1-2): II = +1 Protein (1-2): II = +1 Nuts (0.5): I = +1 Grains (2): II = +1 Good fats: I = +1 Dairy (1): I = +1
			Quality points: 8 Deductions: 0 Food score: 8 **Perfect score!**
A.M. snack: Chocolate banana spinach smoothie	Sometimes you have to break a recipe down into its ingredients to tally.	Veggies: I Fruits: I Beans: Protein: I Nuts: I Grains: Good fats: Dairy:	
Ingredients: 1/3 cup whey protein powder, chocolate flavor 1 cup almond milk 1 frozen banana 1 cup loosely packed spinach leaves			

What I Ate	How to Tally		How to Score
Lunch: Spicy black beans, avocado, cilantro Ingredients: 1 cup black beans 0.5 cups carrots and cilantro 0.5 cups garlic and onions Half an avocado	More than 1 vegetable was needed to reach the recommended 1 cup (and accrue 1 tally mark).	Veggies: I Fruits: I Beans: I Protein: Nuts: Grains: Good fats: Dairy:	
P.M. snack: Carrots and hummus		Veggies: I Fruits: Beans: I Protein: Nuts: Grains: Good fats: Dairy:	

Dinner: Chicken, 1 cup brown rice mixed with 1 tablespoon coconut oil, 1 cup side salad with balsamic vinaigrette	Good fats can be mixed into a variety of other food groups; remember to record them. Vinaigrette is a cost-neutral food item.	Veggies: I Fruits: Beans: Protein: I Nuts: Grains: I Good fats: I Dairy:			
Breakfast: 2 pieces white toast with cottage cheese and strawberry jelly	White bread counts as sugar, so does jelly. This breakfast lost tally marks for fruit and grains and gained deductions	Veggies: Fruits: Beans: Protein: Nuts: Grains: Good fats: Dairy: I Deductions: II	Veggies (4): III Fruits (3): II Beans (1-2): II Protein (1-2): II Nuts (0.5): I Grains (2): Good fats: I Dairy (1): II	= = = = = = = =	0 0 +1 +1 +1 0 +1 0

What I Ate	How to Tally	How to Score
A.M. snack: Chocolate and banana smoothie Ingredients: 1/3 cup whey protein powder, chocolate flavor 1 cup almond milk 1 frozen banana	Without the spinach, this smoothie moves down in quality.	Quality points: 4 Deductions: 3 Food score: 1 Room for improvement
	Veggies: Fruits: I Beans: Protein: I Nuts: I Grains: Good fats: Dairy:	1. Make sure to get veggie points. Adding leafy greens to smoothies and sandwiches is easy. 2. Eat fresh fruits and veggies as snacks. Add them to breakfast. 3. Choose whole grains, never white rice or bread. 4. Except for fresh fruits and veggies, don't exceed serving goals. 5. Use homemade dressing: olive oil mixed with lemon juice, salt, and pepper.

Lunch: Spicy black beans topped with yogurt, avocado, cilantro	Notice the additional dairy serving pushes past the recommended rule in the dairy category of having no more than one	Veggies: I Fruits: I Beans: I Protein: Nuts: Grains: Good fats: I Dairy: I
Ingredients: 1 cup black beans 0.5 cups carrots and cilantro 0.5 cups garlic and onions Half an avocado 1 cup plain yogurt		
P.M. snack: Carrots and hummus		Veggies: I Fruits: Beans: I Protein: Nuts: Grains: Good fats: I Dairy:

What I Ate	How to Tally		How to Score
Dinner: Chicken, 1 cup white rice mixed with 1 tablespoon coconut oil, 1 cup side salad with ranch dressing	We lost the nutrition in rice by choosing white rice over brown, so no points are earned in the grains category. Store-bought dressings cause deductions.	Veggies: I Fruits: Beans: Protein: I Nuts: Grains: Good fats: I Dairy: Deductions: I	

How Do I Know If I Am Eating a High-Quality Diet?

The food score represents diet quality as a number that ranges from -8 to +8. A score of -8 means you are likely not following any of the diet recommendations. You are mainly eating foods on the deductions list. A score of 0 means you are not eating enough healthy foods to outweigh the harm caused by eating unhealthy foods. A score of +8 is the best because it means you matched the recommended diet exactly.

What Should I Know About Diet Quality and Weight Loss?

Most women will find they need a food score of at least 5 to achieve sustainable, healthy weight loss of about 0.5 to 1 pound per week. For some women, even higher quality diets—scores of 6 and 7—will be needed to get weight loss results. Your journal asks you to track what you're eating and give yourself a food score EVERY DAY so you can see what works for you.

Don't I Have to Count Calories?

For the average woman to maintain her weight, she needs to consume between 1600 and 1800 kcal daily. Women older than 50 need about 1600 kcal, while women between 30 and 49 need about 1800 kcal. To lose weight, stay healthy, and prevent diet-busting cravings which lead to overeating, we recommend eating about 1600 kcal daily while gradually increasing your activity level as prescribed in your training plan. This method will create the calorie deficit required to give you weight loss.

Research shows that most of us underestimate the number of calories we eat. Calorie counting is difficult and time consuming. This is why we recommend using a standard cup measure to decide how much of each food category to eat. In the next chapter, we also do the hard work of calorie counting for you by recommending specific meals and snacks based on 200 kcal to 400 kcal per meal.

What Do I Need to Know About Animal Protein Versus Plant Protein?

For the purposes of calculating your food score, we distinguish between animal sources of protein (lean protein), plant sources of protein (beans and nuts), and milk sources of protein (dairy). Each source of protein has a place in a healthy diet. For example, tofu is from soybeans (a plant), so tofu should be tallied as a serving of beans in the food score. On the other hand, eggs come from fowl (animal), so even though eggs traditionally are thought of as a dairy product—and are found next to cheese and yogurt in the grocery store—in the food score, eggs count as lean protein. In the food score, the dairy category is regarded as milk-based products only.

What About Serving Sizes?

One cup of fresh or frozen veggies is the same as 1/2 cup cooked veggies, and 1 cup of fresh or frozen fruit is the same as 1/4 cup dried fruit or 1/2 avocado. When eating baked goods such as a waffle or pancake, use the 1 cup measure for the wet batter to guess how many servings to count.

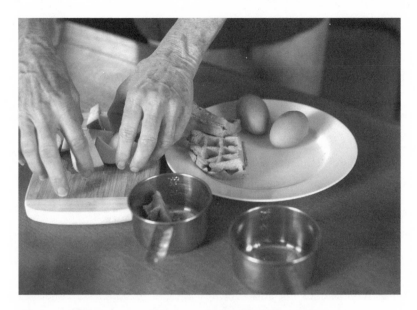

Are There Any Half Points (0.5 Point)?

Yes, there are some foods and drinks that earn 0.5 points when eaten in common portions. You may find it helpful to record half points as dashed lines in your food journal. Make the line solid when you eat another 0.5-point portion.

- 1 scoop (about 1/3 cup) protein powder is about the same as 0.5 point of lean protein

- 1 cup of almond milk is about the same as 0.5 point of nuts

- 1 cup of soy milk is about the same as 0.5 point of beans

- 1 slice of whole-grain bread is about the same as 0.5 point of healthy grains

- 1 egg is about the same as 0.5 point of lean protein

What Is a Healthy Approach to Alcohol?

Alcohol can be enjoyable. Red wine in particular appears to provide some anti-aging benefits believed to be related to a chemical called reservitrol. However, problems with alcohol go under-recognized in our society. Women tend to under-report the amount of alcohol they drink and underestimate the amount of calories in alcoholic beverages. The key to good health, especially when weight loss is a goal, is to consume alcohol in low to moderate amounts with accurate judgment as to the amount in serving sizes. One serving of alcohol is 5 ounces of wine or 12 ounces of beer.

The Rx Eat does not allow for any amount of liquor, and one beer leads to a -1 point deduction.

Women should not consume more than 7 servings of alcohol in one week and never more than 3 servings in one sitting. Avoid getting drunk—it's never good for you.

What About Eggs?

Eggs are a healthy, inexpensive source of protein. Egg yolks are high in cholesterol but do not seem to have much impact on blood cholesterol. You can see we recommend them in the diet as a cheap and healthy source of protein. If you have diabetes or high cholesterol, we recommend eating less than seven eggs in one week.

A Word About Red Meat

Red meat (e.g., steak, pork, venison, goat, salami, ham, sausage) is not part of the Mediterranean diet. You probably noticed that eating red meat hurts your food score. Because eating red meat has been linked to cancer, we actively discourage eating red meat. However, we understand some women have reasons of their own for eating protein in the form of red meat. Keep track of how much red meat you eat in your journal and realize that when you eat it, you get a deduction. If you are not reaching your weight loss goals, consider eating fewer portions or better yet, dropping it altogether.

The Ancient Greeks Ate Full-Fat Dairy and You Should, Too

Contrary to popular belief, recent studies are showing that full-fat dairy products may actually be good for your heart and circulation. They're a good thing to have in a weight loss diet because they help you get the nutrients you need to stay healthy and feel more satisfied after a meal. In short, full-fat dairy helps you stick to your Rx Eat.

Healthy Fats

Healthy fats include olive oil, seed oils, and oils in fatty fish. Your brain, muscles, and joints need these fats to work well. The trouble is that fat is high in calories. That's why the key to weight loss on a diet that includes fat is to eat healthy fats in small amounts. It may also surprise you to learn that butter does not seem to be as bad for your health as was once believed. If you like butter, go ahead and have a little bit. Just make sure to stay below the recommended 3 tablespoons of total fat per day.

A Word About Diet Soda

Even if the soda claims zero calories, research shows women who drink diet soda often gain weight and suffer more heart attacks. The jury is still out as to the reasons for this. Some believe artificial sweeteners play a role. For now, suffice it to say—if the ancient Greeks didn't drink it, neither should you.

What Should I Drink?

Every meal, drink 8 to 10 ounces of water (a big glass) and make sure you drink at least that much between each meal so that every day you drink 6 to 8 glasses of water. You will know you are hydrated enough if you have to pee at least once every two hours or so. Most women find that to do this, they have to carry a re-useable water bottle in their purse and car.

If you don't enjoy plain water, add a splash of fresh lime or lemon slices. You can also make a pitcher of water and toss in diced strawberries or cucumbers. Leave the pitcher in the refrigerator for a couple of hours or overnight to give the water flavor.

Black coffee and unsweetened tea are allowed in this diet and do not change the food score. Both coffee and tea are enjoyable, healthy parts of our own diets. One word of caution: be very careful if you choose to put honey into your drinks. Honey contains about 60kcal per tablespoon, so it's easy to lose track of additional calories.

I'm Known for My Sweet Tooth—What Can I Do?

For someone who loves sweets, and is used to having a lot of sugar in her diet, it takes time to get used to a diet that allows only fruit and honey as sources of sweetness. Be patient with yourself. Remain determined. Know your taste buds can be encouraged to adjust to healthy eating and your palate can be changed. In the meantime, you might be able to soothe your sweet tooth by combining honey with fruit for utmost sweetness. For example, dip frozen grapes or bananas into a tablespoon of honey and enjoy this as a snack. Some flavored whey protein powders (like chocolate) are sweet and can be mixed into smoothies. You can also flavor sparkling water with fresh fruit like strawberries or oranges. A piece of dark chocolate and a glass of wine might do the trick (and won't hurt your food score when enjoyed in small amounts).

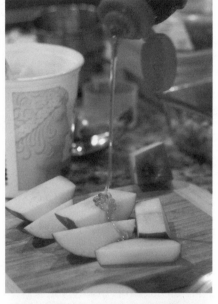

Remember these four steps:

1. Choose foods from the list.

2. Record everything you eat.

3. Tally every time you eat.

4. Score and record your food for the day.

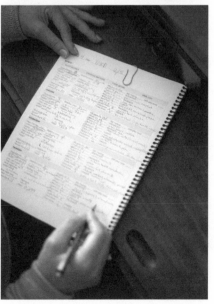

This might seem like a lot. Don't get discouraged if your food score is not always perfect.

Remember, aim for as high a score as you can get. The daily Rx includes the Rx Run-Walk and what you eat, which we call your Rx Eat. Think of your combined Rx Run-Walk and Rx Eat as one complete prescription for health. They work together and you need to follow both to get the results you want!

In the next section, let's put it all together.

Rx Eat—Get Started

In chapter 3, you found the Rx Run-Walk that is right for you. Each of the Rx Run-Walk prescriptions has a matching Rx Eat that tells you how much food within each category of the Mediterranean diet you should eat and how often. The Rx Eat shows you what portion sizes should be based on how food looks on your dinner plate. Most women need to eat at least four times a day. Sometimes five small meals are better.

Consider this before you start:

1. Rx Eat assumes you do not have food allergies. For most women, the full Mediterranean diet consists of eight categories: vegetables, fruits, nuts, beans, whole grains, dairy, lean protein, and good fats. However, if you are allergic to a particular category like nuts or dairy, you will have to avoid it. In this case, your maximum food score will be adjusted to 7. The important thing for you is to watch carefully for a food score that helps you reach your health and weight loss goals.

2. Vegetarians are encouraged to substitute lean protein for eggs (if not vegan) or when not eating eggs; instead proportionately increase portions of the food categories which include protein such as beans, whey protein powder, nuts, and dairy. For example, if you do not eat eggs on a particular day, increase your serving of beans by 1 cup and add +2 to your food score when you've eaten 3 cups of beans. Alter-

natively, you could increase your serving of nuts by 0.5 cup and add +2 to your food score when you've eaten a total of 1 cup of nuts for the day.

3. If you have diabetes or pre-diabetes, Rx Eat assumes you partner with a nutritionist as you do the program.

Just like the Rx Run-Walk prescriptions, the Rx Eat prescriptions build upon one another. Let's look at them now.

In the Rx Eat: Get Started prescription, you eat a total of about 1600 kcal daily divided into four meals. The food you choose should come from each of the eight categories in the assigned amounts. You calculate and record your food score daily, and aim for a score of 6 or better.

R$_X$ Eat — GET STARTED

Ruth Parker, MD and Carmen Mohan, MD
Better Health
Atlanta, GA 30307

Name: _____ Age: _____
Address: _____
Date: _____

R$_X$ Each day, eat 400 kcal at breakfast, lunch, and dinner
PLUS one high quality 200 kcal snack. Aim for a
Food Score of at least 6. Include all of the categories below:

Fresh Vegetables	Fresh Fruits	Beans	Protein	Nuts or Seeds	Grains	Good Fats	Dairy
at least 4 cups	at least 3 cups	1 - 2 cups	1 - 2 cups	up to 0.5 cups	up to 2 cups	up to 0.25	about 1 cup

Indications:

☑ Find my healthy weight

☑ Improve heart health

☑ Improve cholesterol

☑ Control blood sugar

☑ Lower blood pressure

Fruits Grains Dairy Vegetables Protein

source: ChooseMyPlate.gov

Signature *Ruth M. Parker, MD*   *Carmen Patrick Mohan, MD*

What Can I Expect From Rx Eat—Get Started?

When combined with Rx Run-Walk: Get Started, Rx Eat: Get Started was created to help you lose about one pound every four weeks for a total of about 10 to 12 pounds in one year.

R$_X$ Eat — KEEP GOING

Ruth Parker, MD and Carmen Mohan, MD
Better Health
Atlanta, GA 30307

Name: _____ Age: _____
Address: _____
Date: _____

R$_X$ Each day, eat 400 kcal at breakfast, lunch, and dinner PLUS one high quality 200 kcal snack. Aim for a Food Score of at least 6. Include all of the categories below:

Fresh Vegetables	Fresh Fruits	Beans	Protein	Nuts or Seeds	Grains	Good Fats	Dairy
at least 4 cups	at least 3 cups	1 - 2 cups	1 - 2 cups	up to 0.5 cups	up to 2 cups	up to 0.25	about 1 cup

Indications:

☑ Find my healthy weight

☑ Improve heart health

☑ Improve cholesterol

☑ Control blood sugar

☑ Lower blood pressure

source: ChooseMyPlate.gov

Signature *Ruth M. Parker, MD*   *Carmen Patrick Mohan, MD*

In the Rx Eat: Keep Going prescription, you eat a total of 1600 kcal daily divided into four meals. The food you choose should come from each of the eight categories in the assigned amounts. You calculate and record your food score daily, and aim for a score of 6 or better.

What Can I Expect From Rx Eat—Keep Going?

You'll notice Rx Eat: Keep Going is identical to the Rx Eat: Get Started prescription. However, when you combine Rx Eat: Keep Going with the Rx Run-Walk: Keep Going prescription, you will lose about one pound every two weeks or so for a total of about 20 to 30 pounds in one year.

R$_X$ Eat — BURN FAT

Ruth Parker, MD and Carmen Mohan, MD
Better Health
Atlanta, GA 30307

Name: _____ Age: _____
Address: _____
Date: _____

R$_X$ Each day, eat 400 kcal at breakfast, lunch, and dinner PLUS one high quality 200 kcal snack AND one 200 kcal snack 30 minutes after Walk/Run. Aim for a Food Score of at least 6. Include all of the categories below:

Fresh Vegetables	Fresh Fruits	Beans	Protein	Nuts or Seeds	Grains	Good Fats	Dairy
at least 4 cups	at least 3 cups	1 - 2 cups	1 - 2 cups	up to 0.5 cups	up to 2 cups	up to 0.25	about 1 cup

Indications:

☑ Find my healthy weight
☑ Improve heart health
☑ Improve cholesterol
☑ Control blood sugar
☑ Lower blood pressure

source: ChooseMyPlate.gov

Signature *Ruth M. Parker, MD*   *Carmen Patrick Mohan, MD*

With the Rx Eat: Burn Fat prescription, you eat a total of 1600 kcal daily divided into five meals. The food you choose should come from each of the eight categories in the assigned amounts. You calculate and record your food score daily, aiming for a score of 6 or better.

The main difference between the Rx Eat: Burn Fat prescription and the other two programs is the addition of a post-workout snack—a snack to be eaten after your run-walk. Within 30 minutes to an hour after completing your Rx Run-Walk for the day, you should have a 200-kcal snack. Eating this way helps muscles recover from your run-walk, keeping them healthy and strong. The post-workout snack also encourages your body to use excess fat (instead of muscle) when it looks for fuel. You might also feel more energetic by eating more frequently. For all of these reasons, it is extremely important that you are consistent with the way you follow the Rx Eat: Burn Fat prescription.

What Can I Expect From Rx Eat—Burn Fat?

When combined with the Rx Run-Walk: Burn Fat prescription, you will lose about one pound every week or so for a total of about 50 pounds in one year.

Avoid These Traps!

- Don't strive for more weight loss than your program recommends. If you try to restrict the amount of food even more than what's recommended, you will not get the nutrients you need to be healthy. You are also likely to feel hungry most of the time, leading to a miserable experience. Eating too little causes illness and injury. Trust the program and give your body the time it needs to adjust to your new lifestyle. Your goal is to work up to the full Rx Run-Walk and follow its Rx Eat for 30 weeks, then maintain that for at least 3 months. That is how you get the results in weight loss and better health.

- Don't work out on days when you should be resting. Your body needs the rest days to build muscle and strengthen tendons. Over time, stronger, healthier muscles will help you lose weight.

- Don't starve muscles by skipping recommended snacks after your run-walk. Thirty minutes to an hour after you run-walk is the best time for muscles to soak up nutrients. Skipping recommended snacks will lead to low energy, irritability, and weaker muscles.

CHAPTER 5 SETTING YOURSELF UP FOR SUCCESS WITH RX EAT

Sleep Matters! Rx Sleep

Getting enough sleep is key to maintaining a healthy weight, preventing injury, and feeling better. The kind of sleep that protects health is of good quality and lasts for at least 7 uninterrupted hours. We know hardly anyone gets enough good sleep. Being overweight is associated with poor sleep quality and shorter sleep duration. Unfortunately, studies also show that hormonal fluctuations place women at risk for poor sleep quality.

Here's why getting enough good sleep is fundamental to achieving weight loss. Hormones regulate your appetite, your body's response to stress, and how well your body metabolizes the food you eat. When you do not sleep enough, your hormones change in a way that makes you gain weight because lack of sleep makes the following things happen:

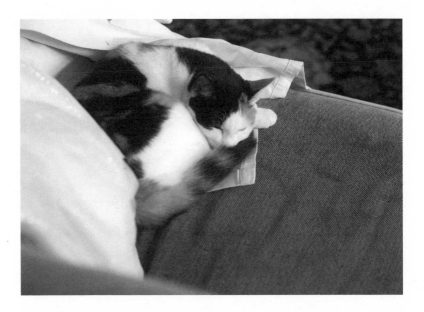

1. You feel hungry.

2. Your body is stimulated to store fat.

3. You feel more stressed and less able to cope.

4. Your will power is reduced.

All of this adds up to mean you eat more calories when you don't get enough sleep and your body puts those extra calories into fat storage.

Here's the good news. When you get enough sleep, you are:

✓ more attentive,

✓ better able to organize, and

✓ more likely to sustain the will power required to make healthy changes.

There's more good news—exercise improves sleep economy. That means women who run-walk get better quality sleep.

Tips for getting better sleep:

    ✓ Go to bed at the same time every night.

    ✓ Get up at the same time every morning.

    ✓ Keep electronic devices out of the bedroom. This includes cell phones, computers, and televisions.

    ✓ Don't let pets sleep in your bedroom.

    ✓ Avoid drinking caffeine after 2:00PM. It'll keep you awake!

    ✓ If you decide to drink alcohol, do so before 8:00PM. All forms of alcohol shorten the sleep cycle.

    ✓ Don't smoke.

    ✓ Avoid napping.

Menopause and Sleep

Forty percent of women experience sleep problems during menopause. But there's good news! Rx Run-Walk will help improve the quality of sleep during menopause.

Sleep Apnea

If you have been told you have a sleeping disorder like obstructive sleep apnea, make sure you use your CPAP machine every night.

R$_X$ Sleep

Ruth Parker, MD and Carmen Mohan, MD
Better Health
Atlanta, GA 30307

Name: _____ Age: _____
Address: _____
Date: _____

℞ Get into bed before 10:00PM every night and sleep for at least 7 hours. For best results, your bedroom should be free of pets and of all digital devices including cell phones, TVs, and computers.

Indications:

☑ Restore bones, joints, and muscles   ☐ Breathe more easily

☑ Improve mood, mental well-being, coping   ☐ Improve cholesterol

☑ Get more restorative sleep   ☑ Control blood sugar

☑ Improve heart health and circulation   ☐ Lower blood pressure

☑ Improve thinking and remembering   ☑ Find my healthy weight

Signature   *Ruth M. Parker, MD*   *Carmen Patrick Mohan, MD*

Moving Matters!

Regardless of which Rx Run-Walk prescription you are following, you should be taking 5,000 to 6,000 steps every day. You should be taking these steps IN ADDITION to doing your Rx Run-Walk. Studies have shown you need to do about 8,000 steps a day to maintain your weight and 10,000 to 12,000 steps a day for weight loss.

Strategies, Tools, and Recipes

Tips for Success With Your Rx Eat: Plan, Plan!

Before you start, try these suggestions:

✓ Create a space for meal planning in your calendar. At the beginning, you will typically need about an hour. Carmen usually does this on Sundays.

✓ Create a space in your calendar for grocery shopping.

✓ Have things you will need on hand: a reusable water bottle, reusable lunch box, and dishwasher-safe containers.

✓ Prepare your household for the new food coming their way. Request their support in improving everyone's health, not just yours.

Following your Rx Eat prescription requires strategic planning on a weekly basis. Here's how to organize your life so you stick to your Rx Eat. **Plan your food and eat only what you planned.**

A Four-Step Plan for Rx Eat Success

Step 1 Plan Every Meal

Look at your work and life schedule. Decide which days you will cook and eat at home and which days you will eat out. Attack the hardest question first—what's for dinner? Plan leftovers, pick-up, or delivery for evenings when your household is busiest.

Generally, Carmen finds the following pattern for a week of dinner planning works well for her busy household of four: two fish meals, one poultry meal, two vegetarian meals, and two meals of leftovers or eating out. She then traces her footsteps back to see if any leftover dinner items can be reused in lunches for the week.

Her lunch patterns include: two lunches from leftovers, one pre-made/ store-bought lunch (e.g., sushi), three sandwiches, and one surprise or new food.

Her breakfast patterns include: one or two make-ahead items (e.g., muffins, yogurt parfaits, breakfast burritos, hard-boiled eggs), two pre-made breakfasts (e.g., cereal and nuts), and three easy-to-make-in-real-time breakfasts (e.g., toast with nut butter).

Write down all of the meals you will eat for the week, including breakfasts, lunches, and snacks. Flip through a recipe book or magazine (Ruth likes *Cooking Light*) looking for meals that appeal to you. Write down the page number next to the meal on your plan for easy reference when you are cooking. Also note where a make-ahead item lies (e.g., pizza dough, marinade sauce, frozen banana, roasted beet, hard-boiled eggs).

As you are planning, use the food score to help you plug holes. For example, go ahead and tally up each day to create a food score. If you are missing a particular food category, review the list to see if there is an easy way to include that category to boost your score for the day. See the table below for ideas. Post the meal plan for the week on the fridge so everyone in your household knows what to expect that week.

It will probably take between 2 to 3 months to develop your go-to meals—meals you discover you enjoy and also are in keeping with your Rx Eat. Save your weekly meal plans so you can recycle the best ones. Carmen has found that doing this consistently over the course of a year allows her to reuse her best meal plans to eat seasonally and locally.

Weekly Meal Planner

For the week of:	Dinner
Breakfast	Monday
M:	
Tu:	
W:	
Th:	Tuesday
F:	
Sat:	
Sun:	
Lunch	Wednesday
M:	
Tu:	
W:	
Th:	Thursday
F:	
Sat:	
Sun:	
Snacks	Friday
M:	
Tu:	
W:	Saturday
Th:	
F:	
	Sunday
Sat:	
Sun:	

Step 2 Create a Grocery List Based on the Meal Plan

Go to the grocery store and only buy food on the list. Use this grocery store overview to plan how you shop:

- It's hard to go wrong in the areas where you find frozen fruits and veggies, fresh fruits and veggies, and nuts. Incorporating fruits and vegetables will be easiest in these zones.

- In the zones that contain dairy, protein, wine, beans, rice, grains, and good fat are where you need to visit to buy items which should be on your list, but you'll have to be looking for particular items to avoid excess sugar, bad fat, and processed foods. You'll have to be careful with the way you choose (don't fall into the red meat trap or buy unhealthy packaged frozen dinners). You'll only need a few items from these zones.

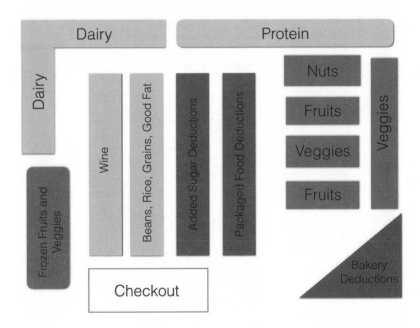

- Finally, the remaining zones are where only deductions lurk. It's easy to buy packaged processed foods that should not be included in your diet. Spend very little time in the these zones if you go down those aisles at all. Generally, you should spend the bulk of your shopping time in the aisles that are closest to the walls of the grocery store.

Step 3 Make Space and Time in Your Daily Schedule for Meal Preparation

Decide when you'll prepare dinner and pack lunches. This is one of the hardest steps because it does take time. Here's another fundamental

GROCERY SHOPPING FOR THE MEDITERRANEAN DIET

LEAFY GREEN VEGETABLES	FRUITS	BEANS	DAIRY
☐ broccoli	☐ apples	☐ black beans	☐ Cheese
☐ spinach	☐ bananas	☐ garbanzo beans	☐ plain yogurt
☐ swiss chard	☐ oranges	☐ hummus	☐ cow milk
☐ kale	☐ berries	☐ kidney beans	☐ _____
☐ collard greens	☐ grapes	☐ navy beans	☐ _____
☐ arugula	☐ melons	☐ pinto beans	☐ _____
☐ _____	☐ pears	☐ soy milk	**LEAN PROTEIN**
☐ _____	☐ pineapples	☐ tofu	☐ eggs
☐ _____	☐ peaches	☐ _____	☐ chicken
	☐ avocado	☐ _____	☐ turkey
OTHER VEGETABLES	☐ raisins	☐ _____	☐ fish
☐ carrots	☐ dates	**WHOLE GRAINS**	☐ almond milk
☐ cucumbers	☐ figs	☐ brown rice	☐ protein powder
☐ garlic	☐ _____	☐ forbidden rice	☐ _____
☐ ginger	☐ _____	☐ wild rice	☐ _____
☐ mushrooms	☐ _____	☐ quinoa	
☐ onions		☐ wheat bread	**GOOD FATS**
☐ peppers	**NUTS**	☐ couscous	☐ olive oil
☐ beets	☐ almonds	☐ wheat pasta	☐ butter
☐ turnips	☐ peanuts	☐ oatmeal	☐ _____
☐ parsnips	☐ cashews	☐ _____	☐ _____
☐ tomatoes	☐ walnuts	☐ _____	
☐ cauliflower	☐ pumpkin seeds	**OTHER STUFF**	**DON'T FORGET**
☐ cabbage	☐ flax seeds	☐ _____	☐ _____
☐ _____	☐ nut butter	☐ _____	☐ _____
☐ _____	(peanut, almond etc)	☐ _____	☐ _____
☐ _____	☐ _____	☐ _____	☐ _____

truth—eating right takes time. At first, cooking and eating differently will require more attention and concentration, but over time, you'll become a pro.

Step 4 Use a Cup Measure to Place Food on Your Dinner Plate

Half of your plate should be non-starchy vegetables, one quarter of it should be protein, and one quarter of it should be healthy grains. Eat meals with others. Enjoy the company. Ban electronics—especially cell phones—at meals. Households that eat together, stay together!

More Tips for Weight Loss and Healthy Eating:

1. Drink 8 ounces of water about 5 minutes before you eat.

2. Drink 4 cups of unsweetened tea daily (green tea is better than black).

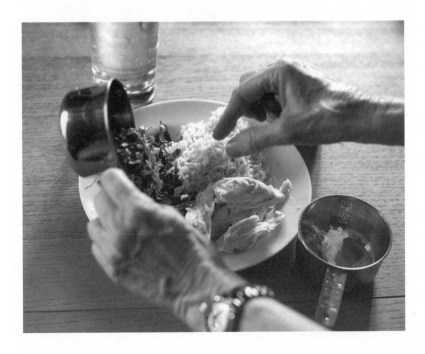

3. Avoid getting hungry. Snack on as many fresh fruits and vegetables as you need to feel good.

4. When you eat out, ask for a to-go container when you order food. Place half of the portion in the container BEFORE you begin eating.

5. When you travel, take a snack with you. An apple and a handful of nuts are easy to carry in your purse. When you arrive at your destination, go grocery shopping as soon as you can even if you're only away from home for a day or two.

Snacks to Always Have Ready

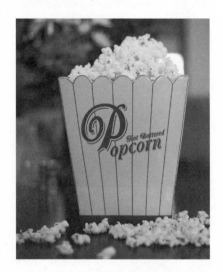

- Hard-boiled eggs

- Hummus

- Fresh fruits and nuts

- Fresh veggies chopped into sticks

- Popcorn

Ways to Score the Veggie Point in the Food Score

- Add a leafy green vegetable to breakfast in an omelette or smoothie. You've already gotten the most important tally mark and the day has just begun!

- Have veggies as part of your snack every day.

- In salads, combine veggies with fruit like citrus, avocado, or berries to make them tasty. Adding cheese crumbles, left over rotisserie chicken pieces, or 1/4 cup of nuts is also a way to make salads more filling.

I'm Eating a Lot of Veggies and Salads. What Can I Put on Them?

Here's a recipe for salad dressing that is in keeping with the Mediterranean diet:

In a small bowl, mix together the following ingredients:

- Juice from 1/2 lemon (Fruit +1)

- 1Tbsp olive oil (Good fat +1)

- 1/8 teaspoon salt

- Sprinkling of pepper to taste

- 2 Tbsp fresh parsley or 1 teaspoon dried basil (Veggie +0.5)

Toss with your favorite veggies for good flavor.

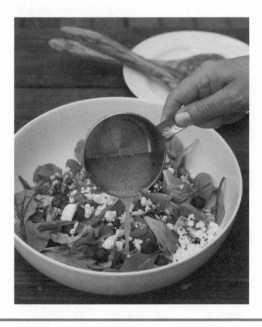

- Some women find they don't like eating green leafy veggies because they are bitter. Try removing some of the bitterness of vegetables (like kale and asparagus) by blanching them. Blanching is a cooking technique where you boil water, then place the cut vegetable into it for one minute and remove. Stop the cooking process by steeping the veggies in ice cold water for another minute.

What If My Significant Other, Kids, or Other Members of My Family Don't Like the Food I Make?

If the foods are new to your household, they can take some time to become popular. Some studies show that a new vegetable has to be

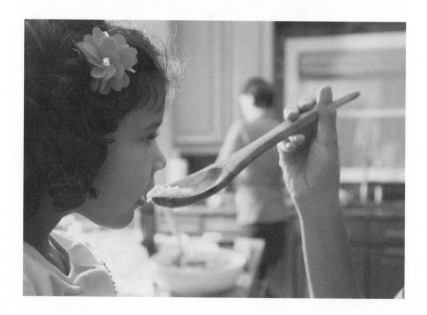

given to children about 15 times before they will be happy eating it. For young children, we recommend the "You don't have to eat it, you only have to try it" approach. Make a deal that eating one spoonful of each new food on the plate is part of a tradition at your table. Say, "Just eat what you like and leave the rest. You don't have to like everything." At the same time, do NOT provide an alternative meal. Adopt this frame of mind: You have taken the time to prepare a nutritious, healthy meal which your family should enjoy as a way to honor you. One household, one meal may seem rigid, but it's one way to lead everyone to healthy living. As they say in Germany "Der Hunger ist der beste Koch" (Hunger is the best cook).

What to Eat During Holidays and Special Occasions?

- Special occasions should be just that—special. These should be one or two days per year, not every other week. Nowadays it seems like every time we turn around, the day is special. Friends' birthdays, children's birthday parties, weddings, Halloween, Valentine's Day, and the winter holidays are just the tip of the iceberg of sugary temptations that make for nothing but food score deductions (and weight gain).

- On the other hand, trying to lose weight during the holidays is not a realistic goal. Doing so makes for misery. Instead of trying to lose weight, your goal should be to enjoy your friends and family without gaining weight. It is okay to sample treats. After the holidays, go back to your plan. Remember, the holidays are only one or two days per year. Decide which days are truly special for you this year. Enjoy those days and then quickly get back to your prescribed food routine.

I've Done Everything You Recommend and I'm Still Not Losing Weight!

- Trying to lose weight can be frustrating and slow going. If it were easy, we wouldn't have written this book.

- Weight loss comes from following your Rx Eat and combining it with your Rx Run-Walk. You will not lose weight if you don't follow both!

- Regardless of whether or not you lose weight, you will gain health with your Rx Run-Walk and Rx Eat.

- In both the Get Started and Keep Going prescriptions, you lose weight from eating good foods in the right amounts while you build your body up to doing more physical activity (and faster weight loss). Make sure you've given your body enough time to adjust (12 weeks) to the Rx Keep Going and Rx Eat. Then, proceed to Rx Run-Walk: Burn Fat and its corresponding Rx Eat prescription.

- Are you getting enough sleep? Remember that sleep is absolutely critical for weight loss. If you are not regularly getting 7 hours of good sleep, your body is working against you in the quest for weight loss.

- Are you at the full dose (week 30) in your Rx Run-Walk? If so, have you been at the full dose for at least 12 weeks? A minimum of 150 minutes of run-walk weekly is required to *maintain* weight.

- You will have to run-walk more than 150 minutes per week if you want to lose weight through exercise. When you are ready, start the Rx Run-Walk: Burn Fat training program and combine it with the Rx Eat: Burn Fat prescription.

- Your Rx Eat requires eating the Mediterranean diet by measuring all food in cups. You should be writing it all down so you have an accurate record of what you are doing. Only after about one month should you lose between 2 and 4 pounds. Are you sure you are recording absolutely everything you eat and drink?

- Review your journal. Where are you receiving deductions? You may need a higher food score to achieve weight loss. Try for scores of 7 or 8. This will mean removing all foods and drinks that lead to deductions.

- If after a month of near-perfect food scores you still haven't seen the scale tip, try eating less frequently. Remove one snack.

- If none of the above solutions works for you, try going old school and start counting calories. Look to see where you are going over the recommended 1600 kcal diet per day. Consider using a smart phone application to count calories like FitDay or MyFitnessPal.

- Show your journal to your doctor and share your concerns. Follow your doctor's advice.

Perfect Score Meal Plans

Breakfasts (400-500 kcal)	Lunches (~400 kcal)	Dinners (400-500 kcal)	Snacks (200-300 kcal)
Breakfast burrito	**Garden salad**	**Baked salmon flavored with lemon**	**Apple and peanut butter**
0.5 cups black beans	2 cups romaine lettuce, cucumbers, carrots, and tomatoes	1 cup arugula	1 apple, sliced
1 egg, scrambled	1 cup navy beans	0.5 cups pomegranate seeds	2 tablespoons peanut butter
1 cup spinach	Olive oil	Goat cheese crumbles	
0.25 cups cheese	Lemon juice	Balsamic vinaigrette	
1 whole-wheat tortilla	Whole-wheat pita bread		
Two-egg omelette	**Hummus, spinach, and cheese sandwich**	**Veggie stir-fry with tofu croutons**	**Raspberry-beet smoothie**
0.5 cups steamed broccoli	Apple	0.5 cups carrots, chopped	1 cup frozen raspberries
Cheddar cheese	Carrot sticks	0.5 cups celery	1 pear
		0.5 cups broccoli	1 beet
		Peanut oil	1 cup almond milk
		0.25 cups ginger	
		Garlic	
		1 cup brown rice	
		0.5 cups tofu croutons	

Multigrain square cereal	Whole-wheat crackers	Baked sweet potato	Cheese and fruit
1 cup cereal	4 whole-wheat crackers	1 cup black beans	0.5 cups cheese, cubed
1 cup almond milk	2 hard-boiled eggs	0.5 cups plain yogurt	4 dates or figs
0.25 cups walnuts	1 cup carrot sticks	Cilantro	
1 cup blueberries	1 orange or apple	Avocado	
		Collard greens, sautéed with onions and garlic in olive oil	

Greek yogurt bowl	Sushi roll	American dinner	Popcorn
1 cup plain whole-fat Greek yogurt	Salmon and avocado rolled in nori, brown rice, and quinoa	1 cup chicken breast	2 cups popcorn with truffle oil
0.25 cups chia seeds	Cucumber slices	Brown rice mixed with coconut oil	
0.25 cups pecans	Pickled ginger	1 cup broccoli, steamed	
1 cup strawberries or blackberries			

Wheat toast	Orange and chicken salad	Bow-tie wheat pasta with greens	Apple and cashew butter
2 slices wheat toast	Garden salad	Kale or collard greens sautéed in 1 Tbsp olive oil with onion, basil, garlic, and sundried tomatoes	1 apple, sliced
0.5 cups cottage cheese	1 cup chicken	Pasta	2 Tbsp cashew butter or nut butter of your choice
Honey	1 Tbsp olive oil and lemon vinaigrette	Capers	
1 cup strawberries	Mandarin oranges	0.5 cups parmesan cheese	
		1 cup navy beans	

Breakfasts (400–500 kcal)	Lunches (~400 kcal)	Dinners (400–500 kcal)	Snacks (200–300 kcal)
Wheat toast	**Turkey sandwich**	**Roasted vegetable platter**	**Wine and chocolate**
2 slices wheat toast	2 slices whole-wheat bread	Brussels sprouts, roasted	1 small piece dark chocolate
Almond butter	2 slices deli turkey	Parsnips, roasted	1 glass (5 ounces) red wine
Banana, sliced	Avocado	Cauliflower, roasted	
	1 apple, sliced	1 cup lentil soup	
		Parmesan cheese	
Oatmeal	**Bento bowl**	**Swiss chard pie**	**Melon**
1 cup oatmeal	Brown rice	1 slice Swiss chard pie	2 cups melon
1 Tbsp honey	Carrots	Cheddar cheese corn muffin	0.25 cups walnuts
Berries	Cucumber		
	Pickled ginger		
	Scrambled egg		
	Tofu		

Smoothie Options (200-400 kcal) to Improve a Food Score

Throw the ingredients into a blender!

Chocolate, Banana, and Spinach Smoothie

- 1/3 cup whey protein powder, chocolate flavor (+1 protein)

- 1 frozen banana (+1 fruit)

- 1 cup spinach leaves (+1 veggie)

- 1 cup almond milk (+1 nut)

Berry Pink Smoothie

- 1 roasted beet, skin removed (+1 veggie)

- 1 pear, cored (+1 fruit)

- 1 cup frozen raspberries (+1 fruit)

- 1 cup almond milk (+1 nut)

- 1/3 cup whey protein powder, vanilla flavor (optional, +1 protein)

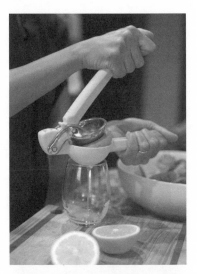

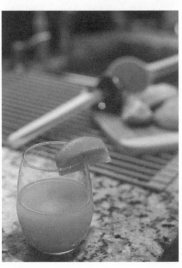

Kale and Coconut Smoothie

- 1 cup coconut water
- 2 kale leaves, stems removed (+1 veggie)
- 1/2 cup plain yogurt (+1/2 dairy)
- 1 tablespoon almond butter (+1 nuts)
- 1 tablespoon honey
- 1 cup ice

Lettuce Drink Smoothie

- 2 leaves romaine lettuce (+1 veggie)
- 1 cup grapes (+1 fruit)
- 1 apple, cored (+1 fruit)
- 1 cup ice
- 1 cup water

Pineapple and Coconut Smoothie

- 8 ounces canned pineapple in juice (unsweetened, +1 fruit)
- 1/4 cup coconut milk (+1 nut)
- 1 cup spinach (+1 veggie)
- 1 cup protein powder, vanilla flavor (optional, +1 protein)

RESOURCES

Cooking Light magazine

CHAPTER 6 ACHIEVE HEALTH GOALS WITH HER PRESCRIPTIONS

Now that you picked out the Rx Run-Walk and Rx Eat that are right for you, let's look at a few very common health goals and see how your **HER Prescriptions** help you with these. We reviewed published scientific studies and called upon national experts to be sure what we present in this section reflects evidence and best medical practice. At the end of each health goal, we suggest a couple of extra resources that we use ourselves.

Many women have more than one specific health goal and will find that their **HER Prescriptions** are helping them address multiple ongoing health needs. For example, we know that there are millions of women with high blood pressure, high cholesterol, and diabetes or pre-diabetes. As we age, we all have aches and pains in bones, muscles, and joints, and we all benefit by finding better ways to cope with everyday life stressors.

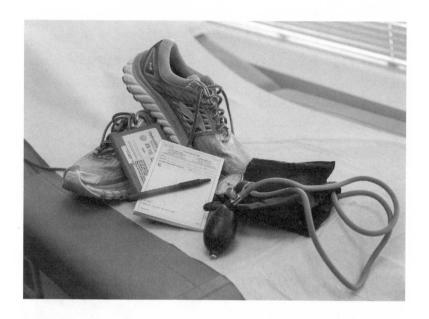

HER Prescriptions are as important for our health as anything we can do. Don't just take our word for it, try it, record your numbers, and prove it to yourself.

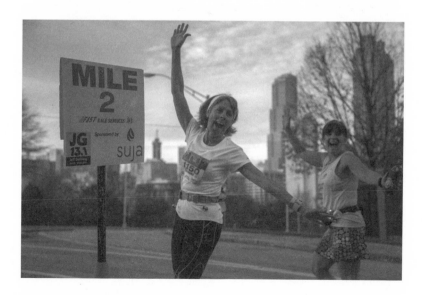

What If My Health Goal Is to Lower My Blood Pressure?

Have you been told you have high blood pressure, hypertension, or elevated blood pressure? If so, this section is especially for you.

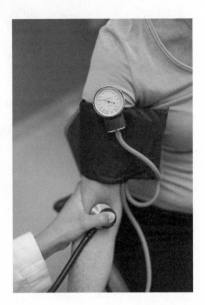

What Are the Facts?

Millions of women have high blood pressure and we know it is associated with heart disease, kidney problems, and strokes. There are good medications to help control blood pressure. In addition to taking medications, Rx Run-Walk can improve your blood pressure.

What Do I Need to Know About HER Prescriptions, Blood Pressure, and Weight Loss?

✓ Taking your Rx Run-Walk in the prescribed way is just as important as taking the other medications you have been prescribed for blood pressure control.

✓ Reaching your full dose Rx Run-Walk will help reduce the risk for stroke by 27%.

✓ Losing just 10% of your starting weight with Rx Eat will lead to a 5mm Hg decrease in your systolic blood pressure (that's the first number in the blood pressure). For every 5% to 10% of additional weight lost, you'll see another meaningful decrease in your blood pressure.

✓ Some women will find that taking their Rx Run-Walk at full dose reduces the number of medications they need. Do NOT stop taking your blood pressure medications without talking to your doctor first.

What Do I Need to Do?

✓ Take your blood pressure medications except your diuretic (water pill that makes you pee) at night. Studies show that taking your blood pressure medications at night better controls your blood pressure when compared to taking medications in the morning.

✓ Follow your Rx Run-Walk and Rx Eat just like you follow dosing instructions for other blood pressure medications. Just like other medications, you should follow the instructions provided for your Rx Run-Walk and Rx Eat, and build up to your full dose carefully and gradually.

✓ REMEMBER: Absolutely NO huffing and puffing when you do your Rx Run-Walk.

What Does It Mean to Self-Monitor?

✓ Take charge! Check your blood pressure every week and record it in your journal.

✓ Before you inflate the cuff, rest for 2 minutes in a seated position with your back supported and your feet flat on the floor. Now, check your blood pressure and record the numbers in your journal. Share your weekly log with your primary care provider.

✓ Take notes and check up on yourself.

✓ Record your blood pressure (BP) in your journal.

✓ Record how you feel in your journal. Work to make this a habit and learn how your body adapts as you become a regular user of your Rx Run-Walk and Rx Eat.

The Doc Box: You Can Still Go Injury-Free

You might have been prescribed one of the following common types of medications: beta-blocker, calcium channel blocker, or diuretic (water pill that makes you pee). These medications impact how you take your Rx Run-Walk. You must warm up gently. In the heat or when you are sweating, be particularly careful—slow down and drink enough water and other fluids. Remember, no huffing and puffing!

Nutrition Tips

1. Toss the canned foods and the salt shaker. Canned beans are usually coated in a lot of salt. If you must eat canned beans, rinse the beans with water before using them.

2. Stay hydrated! Drink 6 to 8 big glasses of water every day.

Resources

**American Heart Association Website,
"Understanding Blood Pressure Readings"**

http://www.heart.org/HEARTORG/Conditions/HighBloodPressure/
GettheFactsAboutHighBloodPressure/Understanding-Blood-
Pressure-Readings_UCM_301764_Article.jsp#.WH5ym7HMxE4

Exercise Is Medicine, "Exercising with High Blood Pressure"
http://www.exerciseismedicine.org/assets/page_documents/EIM%20
Rx%20series_Exercising%20with%20High%20Blood%20Pressure.
pdf

**Patient Education: High Blood Pressure in Adults (Beyond the
Basics) Up-to-Date Patient Sheets**

http://www.uptodate.com/contents/high-blood-
pressure-in-adults-beyond-the-basics?source=search_
result&search=high+blood+pressure&selectedTitle=1%7E101

What If My Health Goal Is to Improve My Heart Health and Circulation?

Have you been told you have heart disease, including any of the following?

- Heart failure (CHF)

- Abnormal heart rhythm

- Atrial fibrillation

- Peripheral vascular disease

- Venous insufficiency

- Circulation problems

- Coronary artery disease (CAD)

- Heart disease

- Heart attack

- Myocardial infarction

If so, this section is especially important for you.

What Are the Facts?

Heart disease is the number one killer of women and it causes 1 in 3 deaths every year. That's scary. Some women feel even more afraid when thinking about starting to exercise when they have been told they have a heart condition. Most women do not understand how vital—meaning absolutely essential—exercise and diet are for heart health. Gentle exercise (i.e., a careful and gradual program) is even

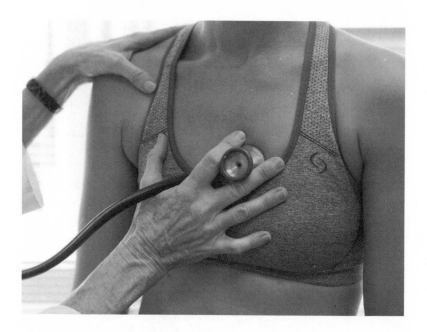

more important when you have a heart or circulation problem. The good news is that following a Rx Run-Walk can make your heart stronger and help you live longer and feel better.

What Do I Need to Know About HER Prescriptions, Heart Health, and Weight Loss?

- ✓ This program has been used successfully for other people like you with heart problems.

- ✓ Losing weight reduces the strain on your heart.

- ✓ Rx Run-Walk prevents and treats heart disease. Following your Rx Run-Walk and Rx Eat is just as important as taking your medications. Doing both is essential to improving your heart function.

- ✓ Taking your Rx Run-Walk at full dose will lower your risk of death from heart disease by at least 20%.

What Do I Need to Do?

- Walk, walk, walk! Take as many breaks as you need. Intensity is your enemy. As you get started with your Rx Run-Walk, your goal is slow and steady not fast and far. No huffing and puffing.

- Use your journal to record how you feel and share it with your doctor.

- Make a plan with your doctor about what to do if you get warning symptoms like chest pain or shortness of breath.

What Does It Mean to Self-Monitor?

- Record how you feel in your journal. Work to make this a habit and learn how your body adapts as you become a regular user of your Rx Run-Walk and Rx Eat.

- For you, it is especially important that you understand and know about your heart and symptoms you have that relate to how your heart is working. Some get short of breath because of their heart health. Some have chest tightness or feel their heart skipping beats or racing. Some may feel completely exhausted, their legs heavy or even painful. If you have been told you have heart disease like heart failure, rhythm problems, coronary artery disease, or circulation problems, or you've had a heart attack, talk to your doctor to be sure you understand how your body signals you about how your heart is functioning. Make a plan with your doctor for what you should look for and what to do.

- At each visit with your doctor, take your journal and your questions!

The Doc Box: You Can Still Go Injury-Free

Start where you are. The training programs are 30 weeks long because it takes this long for your body to adjust and become stronger. In chapter 3, you determined which of the three Rx Run-Walk training programs is right for you. Stay patient and determined. Don't jump ahead. There are no short cuts.

Nutrition Tips

Make sure to eat omega-3s. Omega-3s are a heart-healthy kind of fat. The healthiest way to eat omega-3s is by eating fatty fish like salmon, mackerel, or tuna twice a week. If you don't eat fish, you can get some omega-3s from sources like walnuts, flaxseed, and soybeans. Just be aware that the health benefits aren't as good as eating fish. You can also ask your doctor what dose of fish oil might be good for you as a supplement.

Resources

American Heart Association Exercise and Physical Activity in the Prevention and Treatment of Atherosclerotic Cardiovascular Disease, www.circulationaha.org

What If My Health Goal Is to Improve My Cholesterol?

Have you been told you have one of the following?

- High cholesterol

- Hypercholesterolemia

- High lipids in your blood

- Dyslipidemia

- Hypertriglyceridemia

- Fat in the blood

If so, then this section is especially important for you.

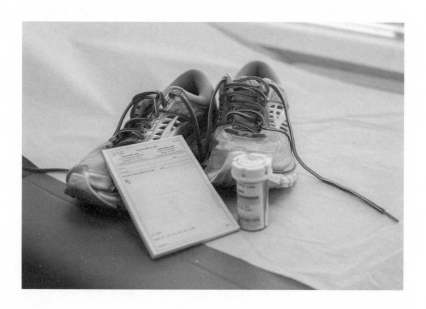

What Are the Facts?

Cholesterol is a fat-like substance in your blood and can build up in the walls of blood vessels. This can lead to heart disease and stroke. You can do a simple blood test to check and follow your cholesterol. Your cholesterol is one of the important health numbers you should know and follow over time because it is associated with heart disease, stroke, and diabetes.

What Do I Need to Know About HER Prescriptions, Cholesterol, and Weight Loss?

- The treatment of high cholesterol is a lifelong process.

- Your Rx Run-Walk and Rx Eat will improve your cholesterol even if you do not lose weight. But, if you are able to lose weight, your cholesterol levels will improve even more.

What Do I Need to Do?

- Think of your Rx Run-Walk and Rx Eat as vital medications for treating your cholesterol.

- After you have been taking your Rx Run-Walk and Rx Eat for at least three months, ask your doctor to recheck your cholesterol. Some women will find that taking their Rx Run-Walk at full dose reduces the number of medications they need. **Do NOT stop taking your cholesterol medication(s) without talking to your doctor first.**

What Should I Put in My Journal About This Condition?

Review your food score in your journal every week. Make sure you are eating fish two times every week. Watch out for deductions. Keep that deduction number below two per week; zero is better!

The Doc Box: You Can Still Go Injury-Free

You may have been given a medication called a statin to help treat your high cholesterol. A small percentage of women who take statins get aches in their muscles when they exercise. If this happens to you, then you might need an even more gradual exercise program. Talk to your doctor if you are worried this might be happening to you. Remember, your prescribed medications work even better when you combine them with your Rx Run-Walk and Rx Eat.

Nutrition Tips

Fish oil—Oily fish, such as mackerel, herring, bluefish, sardines, salmon, and anchovies, contain two important fatty acids, called DHA and EPA. Eating a diet that includes one to two servings of oily fish per week can reduce triglyceride levels (another type of fat in your blood) and reduce the risk of death from heart disease. Fish oil supplements are believed to have the same benefit. Your doctor might recommend that you take a daily fish oil supplement if you are not eating enough fish.

Soy protein—Soy protein contains isoflavones, and these mimic the action of estrogen. A diet high in soy protein can slightly lower levels of total cholesterol, LDL cholesterol, and triglycerides, and raise levels of HDL cholesterol. However, we do not recommend that you replace normal protein sources with soy protein or isoflavone supplements to try to lower your cholesterol level.

Soy foods and food products (e.g., tofu, soy butter, edamame, some soy burgers, etc.) are likely to have beneficial effects on lipids and heart health because they are low in saturated fats and high in unsaturated fats. You will see these listed on your Rx Eat, and can follow guidelines there on eating them.

Resources

Know the Facts About High Cholesterol. National Center for Chronic Disease Prevention and Health Promotion. Division for Heart Disease and Stroke Prevention. http://www.cdc.gov/cholesterol/docs/ConsumerEd_Cholesterol.pdf

What If My Health Goal Is to Breathe More Easily?

Have you been told you have one of the following?

- Bad seasonal allergies

- Asthma

- Chronic obstructive lung disease (COPD)

- Chronic bronchitis

- A problem breathing caused by smoking tobacco

If you have been told you have one of these, then this section is especially for you.

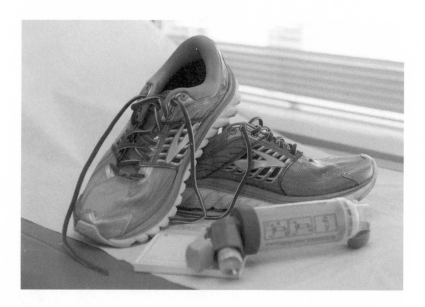

What Are the Facts?

Trouble breathing is commonly caused by asthma, COPD, bad seasonal allergies, or chronic bronchitis. Many women with trouble breathing avoid exercising and because of this, breathing becomes even harder and shortness of breath occurs at even lower levels of activity. When you gradually become more active, you can reverse this and improve your ability to breathe.

What Do I Need to Know About HER Prescriptions, My Breathing, and Weight Loss?

✓ Be aware that stress, anxiety, or a low mood direct your attention to your breathing and make you feel even more breathless.

✓ Achieving your Rx Run-Walk and Rx Eat goals will require patience, determination, and being tuned in to your body's growing ability to adapt and slowly improve over time.

✓ This program has been used successfully for other people like you with breathing problems.

✓ Rx Run-Walk clears sputum from your lungs.

✓ Weight loss makes it easier to breathe.

✓ As you progress with your Rx Run-Walk training program, you will be less short of breath with the same amount of walking.

✓ Women who exercise regularly are able to decrease their need for hospital admissions due to breathing problems.

What Do I Need to Do?

- Walk, walk, walk! Take as many breaks as you need. Intensity is your enemy. As you get started with your Rx Run-Walk training program, your goal is slow and steady, not fast and far. No huffing and puffing at any time!

- Use your journal to record how you feel and share it with your doctor.

- If it is extremely hot or cold outside, or if there is poor air quality, then you should exercise inside by walking on a treadmill.

- Make a plan with your doctor about what to do when you have a flare of your asthma, COPD, or chronic bronchitis. Know how to prevent and manage flare-ups when they happen. If you have been given an inhaler to use, be sure you know how to use it correctly and that you carry it with you.

Record How You Feel in Your Journal

For you, it is especially important that you understand and know about how your breathing problems relate to how your lungs are working. Some women with breathing problems feel very anxious, can't stop coughing, or have difficulty catching their breath. If you have been told you have bad seasonal allergies, asthma, chronic obstructive pulmonary disease (COPD), or chronic bronchitis, be sure you talk to your doctor and understand how your body signals you about how your lungs are functioning.

The Doc Box: You Can Still Go Injury-Free

- If you have been prescribed inhalers or other breathing treatments, make sure to take them as prescribed. Using your inhalers with a spacer device can result in a 20% to 30% increase in the amount of medication delivered to your lungs. If you are not sure how to use your inhalers or a spacer, talk to a health professional like a pharmacist or doctor for help.

- If you have exercise-induced asthma, talk to your doctor about taking a kind of medication called a leukotriene inhibitor which can reduce the symptoms of bronchospasm.

- Bring your rescue inhaler with you when you walk.

If You Smoke

Connect to a support group or program to help you quit.

Resources

Exercising With Chronic Obstructive Pulmonary Disease (COPD), Exercise is Medicine. www.exerciseismedicine.org

Exercising With Asthma, Exercise is Medicine. www.exerciseismedicine.org.

What If My Health Goal Is to Control My Blood Sugar?

Have you been told you have pre-diabetes or diabetes? If so, then this section is especially for you.

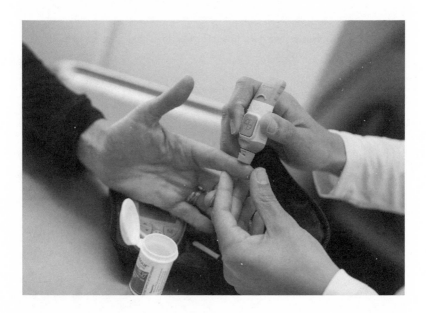

What Are the Facts?

Rx Run-Walk has a key role to play in both preventing and treating blood sugar problems. In fact, Rx Run-Walk can help prevent diabetes-related problems with your nerves and kidneys. These benefits of Rx Run-Walk start the moment you walk out of the door and continue to grow as you work up to the fully prescribed dose of 150 minutes total per week. For example, on the day you run-walk, your blood sugars will be better.

What Do I Need to Know About HER Prescriptions, My Blood Sugar, and Weight Loss?

You can make your blood sugar normal by losing 10% of your body weight using Rx Eat and full dose Rx Run-Walk: Keep Going. In other words, weight loss AND following Rx Run-Walk: Keep Going can markedly improve your diabetes.

What Does It Mean to Self-Monitor?

✓ What and how you eat is especially important because it directly affects your blood sugar control. You have an important role in your own medical care, and monitoring your blood sugar is an opportunity for you to take control of your health.

✓ Record everything you eat and drink honestly and accurately in your journal.

✓ Check your blood sugar in the morning before breakfast and record it in your journal. If it is below 80, eat breakfast before you run-walk. If you feel like your blood sugar might be dropping during your run-walk, eat a piece of fruit or a couple of hard candies. You will become the expert on how your body responds to increasing your exercise.

✓ If your doctor asks you to check your blood sugar two hours after your biggest meal each day, there is space for you to record blood sugar numbers in your journal.

✓ Review your journal entries with your doctor. Ask if any changes to your diabetes medications (including insulin if you use it) are needed.

✓ Partner with a diabetes educator or a dietician to create weekly meal plans.

What Do I Need to Do?

✓ Think of your Rx Run-Walk and Rx Eat as vital treatment for diabetes.

✓ Show your doctor your Rx Run-Walk training program. Ask the following questions:

✓ When should I take my prescription medicine(s)?

✓ Should I eat before physical activity or after?

✓ What should I do if I have low blood sugar during physical activity?

✓ Make a plan with your doctor about what to do if you get symptoms of low blood sugar like feeling shaky or light-headed.

✓ After you have been taking your Rx Run-Walk and Rx Eat for at least three months, ask your doctor to recheck your hemoglobin A1c. Some women will find that taking their Rx Run-Walk at full dose reduces the number of medications they need. Do NOT stop taking your medication(s) without talking to your doctor first about this.

Resources

National Institute of Diabetes and Digestive and Kidney Diseases, Diabetes and Physical Activity. https://www.niddk.nih.gov/healthinformation/diabetes/diabetes-physical-activity

Exercising With Type 2 Diabetes, Exercise is Medicine. http://exerciseismedicine.org/assets/page_documents/EIM%20Rx%20series_Exercising%20with%20Type%202%20Diabetes_2.pdf

American Diabetes Association, Print on-demand materials. http://professional.diabetes.org/search/site?f%5B0%5D=im_field_dbp_ct%3A32&retain-filters=1

What If My Health Goal Is to Restore My Bones, Joints, and Muscles?

Have you been told you have vitamin D deficiency, osteoarthritis, osteoporosis, or had a joint replacement? If you have, then this section is especially for you.

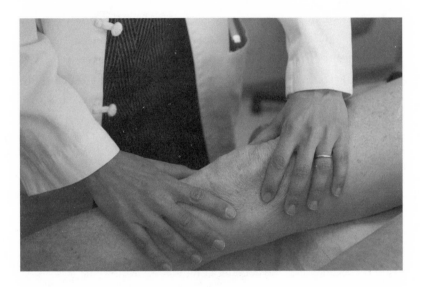

Osteoarthritis: What Are the Facts?

Osteoarthritis, which results from wear and tear on the joint, is the most common cause of joint pain. If we live long enough, we will probably all have osteoarthritis. About one-fourth of all people over age 55 have pain in their knees on most days and most of these people have osteoarthritis. Although not the same for everyone, osteoarthritis tends to be more severe as we age. Many women with joint aches or pains avoid exercising and because of this, moving becomes even harder and at even lower levels of activity. Gradually becoming more active can reverse this, improve your mobility, and actually help to decrease your pain and stiffness. Bones and muscles rely on each other and both require regular use, especially when joints ache and hurt.

What Do I Need to Know About HER Prescriptions, Osteoarthritis, and Weight Loss?

Being overweight and female are risk factors for osteoarthritis of the knees and hips. Exercise with osteoarthritis can be hard and painful and often causes women to be less active. The lack of exercise makes joints stiffer and the surrounding muscles weaker. This leads to the vicious cycle of being even less active. Understand and believe that you can break this cycle. Though you may be taking medications for pain, the Rx Run-Walk will actually restore the health and integrity of painful joints and weak bones and muscles. Your Rx Run-Walk can decrease joint swelling and pain and improve the function of bones, muscles and joints. The key is to gradually start walking using the training program and stay determined to get the benefits.

When you lose weight, you lighten the work of your knees and hips. Weight loss enhances the benefits of regular Rx Run-Walk.

What Do I Need to Do?

- Get started and stay determined. The training program will gently increase your activity level.

- Talk to a fitness coach or physical therapist about weight training. You can often find a professional who can design a weight-training program for you at your gym or YMCA. Personal coaching for weight training is often included with your gym membership.

- Combine your Rx Run-Walk with your Rx Eat to lose 0.5 to 1 pound weekly and keep going until your joints feel good. Target a normal body mass index of between 21 and 25, and plan to reach this goal with slow, steady determination and a plan.

- If you are especially bothered by a certain joint, consider writing down a pain score of 1 to 10 in your journal. Every 4 weeks, look back in your journal to see how the pain score changes. This can be very useful in keeping you motivated.

The Doc Box: You Can Still Go Injury-Free – Osteoporosis

- Osteoporosis, a loss of bone, is a serious concern for women especially as they age. Regular walking and a healthy diet improve the health of bones and muscles throughout life. Walking prevents bone loss because it encourages bone formation, stronger muscles, and better balance. These benefits reduce the chance of falling and breaking a bone.

- This program has been used successfully for other people like you with joint, muscle, and bone problems. This is because bones are designed to support our weight. Bones, especially those of women, require movement and holding weight to be strong. In fact, sitting is the worst thing we do for our bones.

- A regular habit of walking is important to decrease the bone loss that happens in everyone with aging. Walking in a way that significantly increases pain tends to be counterproductive. The use of a cane or hiking staff in the hand opposite the painful joint unloads the hip or knee significantly, and most people can significantly increase the distance of walking before pain becomes limiting by doing so. The cane can therefore be a very useful tool to increase comfortable walking for exercise.

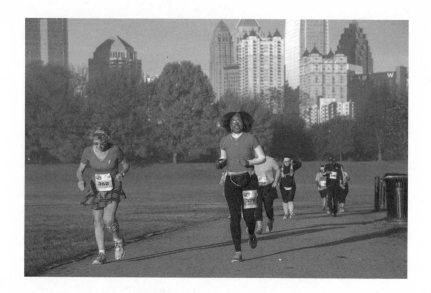

What If I Had a Joint Replacement?

If you have had a joint replacement, to get full benefit of the new joint, you will need to follow the Rx Run-Walk and Rx Eat to get to the full dose of walking and achieve a normal weight with a body mass index (BMI) of 21 to 25.

What If I Was Told I've Got Bone on Bone?

Over time, with repeated use and especially injury, the cushion in the joint space gets smaller. This cushion is called the articular cartilage and sits between the bones of the joint. Even when the bones in a joint contact each other (bone on bone) it is important to understand that your pain and ability to function will likely improve as you move toward your ideal body weight with Rx Eat. For most people, an ideal body weight is a BMI of 21 to 25. It is especially important that you start a weight training program (see below). If you have a joint that is red, swollen, and warm to the touch, you should be evaluated by your doctor. Often times, putting an ice pack on the joint twice a day will help soothe a flare of arthritis. In other words, the vast majority of women will feel better and their joints will be less stiff as they progress through the program. That doesn't mean it will never hurt. It means that you must use pain as your guide.

What If I Have an Old Injury That Causes Aches and Pains?

You can still go, and will find that regularly following your Rx Run-Walk and charting your progress will prove that bothersome aches and pains can improve with regular exercise and weight loss. Our bodies are made to be and stay active!

Bone Health and Joint Pain Improves With Weight Training

No matter the problem with your bones or joints, it can improve with weight training. Especially for those in the Get Started program, the key is to find the exercise activities that provide the most exertion with the least amount of increased pain. A list of activities that work for many people with joint pain includes things like stationary biking or pool exercises. An excellent way for a woman with hip or knee pain to aerobically condition at a high level is with weights. Weight training in this setting should be with lighter weights and high repetitions without resting between sets. Use the machines that do not increase joint pain even if you are limited to working only the upper extremity. With this method it easy to push the heart rate into an aerobic zone without increasing joint pain.

Nutrition Tips

- Vitamin D is essential for bone health. Run-walk outside so you get natural sunlight exposure as often as the weather permits.

- Ask your doctor if you need to take vitamin D supplements.

- Your Rx Eat will give you adequate calcium, but check with your doctor to see if you need more calcium.

Resources

Exercising with Osteoarthritis, Exercise is Medicine. http://exerciseismedicine.org/assets/page_documents/EIM%20Rx%20series_Exercising%20with%20Osteoarthritis.pdf

Exercise and Bone and Joint Conditions, American College of Orthopedic Surgery. http://orthoinfo.aaos.org/topic.cfm?topic=a00100

What If My Health Goal Is to Improve My Mood, Mental Well-Being, and Coping?

Do you have anxiety, seasonal affective disorder, depression, grief, or troubles with smoking, drugs, or alcohol use? If so, this section is especially for you.

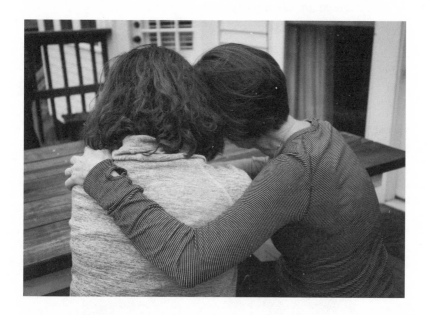

What Are the Facts?

When mental well-being is at risk, learning how to keep yourself motivated and active using Rx Run-Walk is one of the biggest gifts you can give yourself. Knowing the following facts will help you see you are not alone:

- Between the ages of 15 to 55, women are much more likely than men to find that their moods shift with the seasons. You may hear this referred to as seasonal affective disorder.

- While each woman's experience is her own, mood swings are common throughout our lives. Menstrual cycles, pregnancy, the postpartum period, and menopause each have a distinct influence on a woman's mood.

- Women are twice as likely as men to have depression. Forty percent of women will have a depressive episode at some point in their life.

- Grief, loss, and worries about our children and families weigh us down.

Regular exercise is a vital prescription across all ages for women. It gets you outside in the sunlight and among people, and helps you learn to lead with your heart with a smile on your face and find the wind at your back.

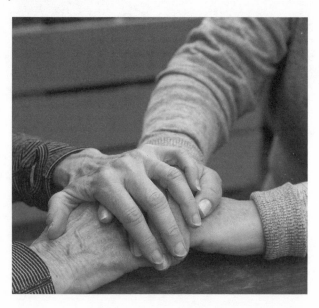

What Do I Need to Know About HER Prescriptions, Mental Well-Being, and Weight Loss?

- The main symptom of depression is fatigue or feeling tired, so getting started is usually the biggest hurdle. Once you regularly run-walk, you're almost half as likely to develop depression.

- Evidence shows that run-walk programs improve anxiety and depression. Your mood, self-esteem, and stress level all get better with regular exercise.

What Do I Need to Do?

✓ Get at least 7 hours of sleep every night. Sleep helps improve mood.

✓ Longer walk sessions are especially important for mental well-being. Getting into the habit and sticking to your routine is especially important.

✓ Studies show that connecting with others who run-walk is essential for getting started and staying committed to reach the full dose of your Rx Run-Walk. Finding a partner or walking group or taking your dog with you can often improve your chances of getting started and keeping going.

✓ Work up to and maintain longer run-walk sessions. Studies show that depression improves at the full dose reached in the Rx Run-Walk: Burn Fat. If you have depression, you should aim to progress through the training programs as you are able and eventually reach the full dose of miles in the Rx Run-Walk: Burn Fat.

✓ Long-term regular exercise lowers anxiety. To fully treat anxiety with the Run-Walk program, aim to complete the Rx Run-Walk: Burn Fat. Maintain it and set gradual fitness goals that extend beyond it. This takes time, determination, and imagination.

How Can I Find a Walking or Running Group?

• Search the web using these keywords "walking for fitness meet-up" followed by your city.

• Check with your human resources department to see if your employer offers walking groups as part of their wellness program.

• Your health insurer or health clinic might also have a list of community resources.

• You can find a list of Galloway Running Groups for over 100 cities at http://www.jeffgalloway.com/training-groups/list-of-cities

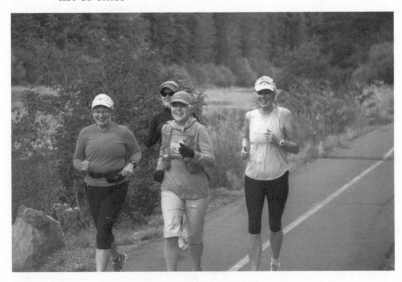

Journal: Especially Important for You!

Use your journal to understand yourself and your habits around Rx Run-Walk, Rx Eat, and the company you keep. Note where you have successes and how success relates to where you run-walk, what you eat, and who you were with, and become an expert at setting yourself up for success. This takes time, patience, and determination.

There is a reflection section in the journal in which you are asked to complete the sentence "I feel…" Make sure you fill out that section regularly and look back every now and then to see how you are doing.

What Do I Need to Know About Smoking, Drugs, and Alcohol Use?

Use of any amount of tobacco and overuse of alcohol continue to be common problems; both negatively influence your mood. Remember your Rx Eat addresses everything you eat and drink. Finding a way to stop all use of tobacco and limit alcohol is part of your Rx Eat. Your Rx Run-Walk and Rx Eat are vital components of your overall approach to treating addiction. If you stick to the amount of alcohol that is allowed in your Rx Eat, you will not be drinking alcohol at a dangerous level.

Resources

Exercising With Anxiety and Depression, Exercise is Medicine http:// exerciseismedicine.org/assets/page_documents/EIM%20Rx%20 series_Exercising%20with%20Anxiety%20and%20Depression_2. pdf

John J Ratey. *Spark: The revolutionary new science of exercise and the brain.* January 2013.

Robert Waldinger. What makes a good life? Lessons from the longest study on happiness. http://www.ted.com/talks/robert_waldinger_ what_makes_a_good_life_lessons_from_the_longest_study_on_ happiness/transcript?language=en

Frequently Asked Questions

If you have a question not covered in this section, we want to hear from you! Please contact us through our website www. HERprescriptions.com.

Why do so many women who lose weight gain it back?

Did you know every year after age 35, a woman's metabolism slows down such that she is destined to gain 0.5 to 1 lbs per year? It's unfair but true. Add in another 0.5 to 1 lbs per year for sleeping less than seven hours a night, and that's a two-pound weight gain per year before we can even blink. Regained weight is most often related to no longer following a careful Rx Run-Walk and Rx Eat. In addition, your body does reset—it becomes more efficient in the way it uses the calories you eat. To offset the silent weight creep, women must get and stay active, eat well, and sleep enough.

What do I do if I can't do my Rx Run-Walk on the scheduled day?

The specific Rx Run-Walk days were chosen because based on our experience, most women have been successful at regularly doing Rx Run-Walk on that particular schedule. Our preference is that you think outside the box and move other priorities around to make room for Rx Run-Walk as the schedule is prescribed. If due to unusual circumstances, you are going to miss just one day, but the regular schedule usually works for you, go ahead and move the Run-Walk to a rest day that is convenient for that week. Then go back to the regular schedule.

If you are just not able to make the regular schedule work for you, here are some rules of thumb:

- Run-walk at least four days per week.

- Always arrange for a rest day after a hard run-walk day.

- Do not run-walk more than two days in a row. You need a rest day after two days of run-walk.

- Do not have a rest day on more than two days in a row.

Should I run when I have a cold?

There are so many individual health issues with a cold that you must consider your unique situation to find the answer that's right for you. There are many infections that initially seem to be a normal cold but are not. If you feel bad enough to stay in bed, you might need to call your doctor's office. If you feel well enough to consider doing Rx Run-Walk, it's likely okay to do so. Here are some red flags (i.e., reasons to skip Rx Run-Walk for the day:

✗   Don't do your Rx Run-Walk for the day if you have a fever, chills, or muscle aches.

✗   Don't do your Rx Run-Walk if you have breathing problems that do not improve with your regular medications. If you have to use your rescue inhaler more than once, don't do Rx Run-Walk, call your doctor.

✗   Don't do your Rx Run-Walk if you are dizzy, or having chest pain or difficulty thinking. Be in touch with your doctor.

What if I missed doing my Rx Run-Walk for a week?

If you have been regularly taking your Rx Run-Walk (for at least 12 weeks), you can probably just pick up your schedule where you left off. Studies have shown that you can maintain conditioning even when you don't run-walk for five days in a row. Surely you want to continue regular run-walks if you can, but staying injury-free has an even higher priority.

How do I know that I am injured?

If you feel any of the three signs of injury listed here, you should stop your run-walk immediately and take some extra rest days (at least two days in a row). Continuing to do the same exercise that irritated the tendon or muscle at early stages of an injury creates a dramatically worse injury, even during one workout. If you take 2 to 3 days off at the first symptom, you may avoid having to stop exercise for 2 to 3 months by trying to push through the pain. It is always safer to err on the side of taking more time off when you first notice one of the following signs:

1. Inflammation—any type of swelling, redness, or warmth

2. Loss of function—the injured area doesn't work correctly

3. Pain—the kind that doesn't go away when you rest for a few minutes

How do I start back when I've had time off?

The longer you've been away from Rx Run-Walk, the slower you must return.

Less than 2 weeks off. You will feel like you are starting over again but should come back quickly. Let's say that you are at week 10 in your training program but had to take 10 days off. Start back at week 2 for the first week. If all is well, skip to week 4 for the second week. If that works well, gradually (i.e., over the next 2 to 3 weeks) transition back to the week 10 schedule you were using before you had your layoff. If you were already taking the week 30 dose—considered your full dose of Rx Run-Walk—start back at week 20 and gradually work your way back from there based on how you feel.

14 days to 29 days off. You will feel like you are starting over again and it will take you longer to get it all back. Within 5 to 6 weeks you should be back to normal. Start at week 1 of your Rx Run-Walk training program. If there are no aches, pains, or lingering fatigue, then use the training schedule but skip every other week. If you feel good after doing the week 10 schedule, transition back into what you were doing before the layoff.

One month or more off. If you have not done your Rx Run-Walk for a month or more, start over again like a beginner. Reread chapter 3 and use the questions there to find the Rx Run-Walk that's right for you. Then start at week 1 of your new training program.

CONCLUSION

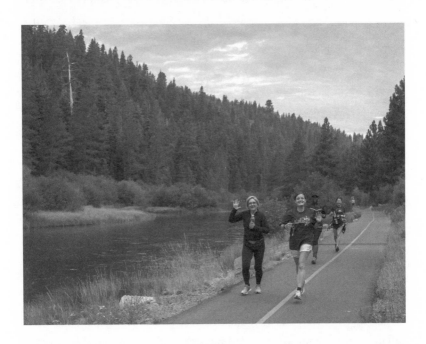

You've seen her run past you on the street. She's got long muscular graceful legs and a smile on her face. Whether young, middle age, or older, she inspires you and many around her. Women are underappreciated brokers of health. The choices women make for themselves and their families really do inspire and influence not just their own health, but the health of many others. From childhood to adolescence, from motherhood to menopause, well into the ninth decade and beyond, women who are run-walkers become health brokers for families and neighbors, as they provide inspiration to the world.

In this book we embrace the philosophy of prescribing run-walk, sleep, and what you eat like a medicine. We walked you through the steps of becoming one of the women in the park, actively engaged with your head up high and confident that taking these prescriptions seriously is good for you, your family, and the people around you. Through the combined lenses of coaching and practicing medicine, we repeatedly see women who have been transformed by choosing to take these prescriptions seriously.

You can do this! You can do this safely. You can do it even if your knees hurt. You can do it even if you are busy, overweight, or overwhelmed. Stay determined. Stay positive and let this guide help you one step at a time.

Remember that you can download and print all the figures, tables, and journal pages from this book at our website, www.HERprescriptions. com. We want to hear from you. If you have questions, need suggestions, or want to share your success story, please visit our website.

Enjoy and smile—join others choosing to lead with our hearts, our heads held high, and the wind at our backs!

CONTENT SOURCES

Chapter 1 Journal

WikiHow. "How to Measure Your Waist." *WikiHow.* Accessed February 27, 2017. www.wikihow.com/Measure-Your-Waist.

Chapter 2 Set Yourself Up for Success with Rx Run-Walk

Mayo Clinic. "Kegel Exercise How-To Guide for Women." *Mayo Clinic.* Accessed February 27, 2017. www.mayoclinic. org/healthylifestyle/womens-health/in-depth/kegel-exercises/art-20045283.

Subak LL, Wing R, West DS, et al. Weight Loss to Treat Urinary Incontinence in Overweight and Obese Women. *The New England journal of medicine.* 2009;360(5):481-490. doi:10.1056/ NEJMoa0806375.

Chapter 3 Find the Rx Run-Walk That's Right for You

Physical Activity Guidelines Advisory Committee. *Physical Activity Guidelines Advisory Committee Report, 2008.* Washington, DC: U.S. Department of Health and Human Services. 2008.

Chapter 4 You Gotta Eat

American Diabetes Association. "Standards of Medical Care in Diabetes—2016 Abridged for Primary Care Providers." Clinical Diabetes 34, no. 1 (2016): 3-21

Da Boit, M. "Sex differences in the effect of fish oil supplementation on the adaptive response to resistance exercise training in older people: a randomized control trial." American Journal of Clinical Nutrition (2016). [Epub ahead of print]

Estruch, R. et al. "Primary Prevention of Cardiovascular Disease with a Mediterranean Diet." New England Journal of Medicine (2013):1279-1290.

Mozaffarian, D. et al. "Dietary and Policy Priorities for Cardiovascular Disease, Diabetes, and Obesity: A Comprehensive Review." Circulation 133, no. 2 (2016): 187-225.

Pimpin, L. et al. "Is Butter Back? A Systematic Review and Meta-Analysis of Butter Consumption and Risk of Cardiovascular Disease, Diabetes, and Total Mortality." PLoS One 11, no. 6 (2016).

Slawson, D.L., N. Fitzgerald, and K.T. Morgan. "Position of the Academy of Nutrition and Dietetics: The role of nutrition in health promotion and chronic disease prevention." Journal of the Academy of Nutrition and Dietetics 113, no. 7 (2013): 972-979.

Thorning, T.K., et al. "Milk and dairy products: good or bad for human health? An assessment of the totality of scientific evidence." Food & Nutrition Research (2016).

Evidence linking diet soda to cardiovascular events:

Vyas, A., L. Rubenstein, J. Robinson, et al. "Diet Drink Consumption and the Risk of Cardiovascular Events: A Report from the Women's

Health Initiative." Journal of General Internal Medicine 30, no. 4 (2015): 462-468.

Evidence linking moderate coffee consumption to lower CVD risk:

Ding, M., S.N. Bhupathiraju, A. Satija, R.M. van Dam, F.B. Hu. "Long-Term Coffee Consumption and Risk of Cardiovascular Disease: A Systematic Review and a Dose-Response Meta-Analysis of Prospective Cohort Studies." Circulation 129, no. 6 (2014): 643-659.

Chapter 5 Setting Yourself Up for Success with Rx Eat

Lambiase, M.J., K.P. Gabriel, L.H. Kuller, K.A. Matthews. "Sleep and Executive Function in Older Women: The Moderating Effect of Physical Activity." The Journals of Gerontology Series A: Biological Sciences and Medical Sciences 69, no. 9 (2014): 1170-1176.

Montgomery, P. and J. Dennis. "Physical exercise for sleep problems in adults aged 60+." Cochrane Database of Systematic Reviews 4 (2002).

Shechter, A. "Obstructive sleep apnea and energy balance regulation: A systematic review." Sleep Medicine Reviews (2016). [Epub ahead of print]

Sternfeld. B., K.A. Guthrie, K.E. Ensrud, et al. „Efficacy of Exercise for Menopausal Symptoms: A Randomized Controlled Trial." Menopause 21, no. 4 (2014): 330-338.

Ward-Ritacco, C.L. et al. "Feelings of energy are associated with physical activity and sleep quality, but not adiposity, in middle-aged postmenopausal women." Menopause 22, no. 3 (2015): 304-311.

Xiao, Q., F. Gu, N. Caporaso, C.E. Matthews. "Relationship between sleep characteristics and measures of body size and composition in a nationally-representative sample." BMC Obesity 3 (2016): 48.

Yang, P.Y., K.H. Ho, H.C. Chen, M.Y. Chien. "Exercise training improves sleep quality in middle-aged and older adults with sleep problems: a systematic review." Journal of Physiotherapy 58, no. 3 (2012): 157-163.

Chapter 6 Achieve Health Goals with HER Prescriptions

Falk, N. et al. "Medications for Chronic Asthma." American Family Physician 94, no. 6 (2016): 454-462.

Peat, G., R. McCarney, P. Croft. "Knee pain and osteoarthritis in older adults." Annuals of Rheumatologic Disease 60, no. 2 (2001): 91-97.

APPENDIX

My Progress Week By Week

	Number of days slept ≥7 hours	Resting heart rate	Blood pressure	Fasting blood glucose	Total distance run-walk	Number of days with a food score ≥6	Weight (lbs)	Fat %
Starting line								
Week 1								
Week 2								
Week 3								
Week 4								
Week 5								
Week 6								
Week 7								
Week 8								
Week 9								
Week 10								
Week 11								
Week 12								
Week 13								

	Week 14	Week 15	Week 16	Week 17	Week 18	Week 19	Week 20	Week 21	Week 22	Week 23	Week 24	Week 25	Week 26	Week 27	Week 28	Week 29	Week 30

SLEEP METRICS	EXERCISE MATTERS	MEALS
Monday		
Sleep estimate:_____ continuous/uninterrupted	Run-walk (min): _____	Breakfast
	Steps: _____	AM snack
Quality: _____		Lunch
Time I got in bed: _____		PM snack
Time I woke up: _____		Dinner
Tuesday		
Sleep estimate:_____ continuous/uninterrupted	Run-walk (min): _____	Breakfast
	Steps: _____	AM snack
Quality: _____		Lunch
Time I got in bed: _____		PM snack
Time I woke up: _____		Dinner
Wednesday		
Sleep estimate:_____ continuous/uninterrupted	Run-walk (min): _____	Breakfast
	Steps: _____	AM snack
Quality: _____		Lunch
Time I got in bed: _____		PM snack
Time I woke up: _____		Dinner
Thursday		
Sleep estimate:_____ continuous/uninterrupted	Run-walk (min): _____	Breakfast
	Steps: _____	AM snack
Quality: _____		Lunch
Time I got in bed: _____		PM snack
Time I woke up: _____		Dinner

Starting Line Report Card

HEALTH NUMBERS	REFLECTIONS
Weight: _____	I feel...
Waist: _____	
Body fat % _____	
BP: _____ / _____	What works well for me?

Friday

Sleep estimate:_____ continuous/uninterrupted Quality: _____ Time I got in bed: _____ Time I woke up: _____	Run-walk (min): _____ Steps: _____	Breakfast AM snack Lunch PM snack Dinner

Saturday

Sleep estimate:_____ continuous/uninterrupted Quality: _____ Time I got in bed: _____ Time I woke up: _____	Run-walk (min): _____ Steps: _____	Breakfast AM snack Lunch PM snack Dinner

Sunday

Sleep estimate:_____ continuous/uninterrupted Quality: _____ Time I got in bed: _____ Time I woke up: _____	Run-walk (min): _____ Steps: _____	Breakfast AM snack Lunch PM snack Dinner

Weekly Meal Planner

For the week of:	Dinner
Breakfast	Monday
M:	
Tu:	
W:	
Th:	Tuesday
F:	
Sat:	
Sun:	
Lunch	Wednesday
M:	
Tu:	
W:	
Th:	Thursday
F:	
Sat:	
Sun:	
Snacks	Friday
M:	
Tu:	
W:	Saturday
Th:	
F:	
	Sunday
Sat:	
Sun:	

GROCERY SHOPPING FOR THE MEDITERRANEAN DIET

LEAFY GREEN VEGETABLES
- ☐ broccoli
- ☐ spinach
- ☐ swiss chard
- ☐ kale
- ☐ collard greens
- ☐ arugula
- ☐ _____
- ☐ _____
- ☐ _____

OTHER VEGETABLES
- ☐ carrots
- ☐ cucumbers
- ☐ garlic
- ☐ ginger
- ☐ mushrooms
- ☐ onions
- ☐ peppers
- ☐ beets
- ☐ turnips
- ☐ parsnips
- ☐ tomatoes
- ☐ cauliflower
- ☐ cabbage
- ☐ _____
- ☐ _____
- ☐ _____

FRUITS
- ☐ apples
- ☐ bananas
- ☐ oranges
- ☐ berries
- ☐ grapes
- ☐ melons
- ☐ pears
- ☐ pineapples
- ☐ peaches
- ☐ avocado
- ☐ raisins
- ☐ dates
- ☐ figs
- ☐ _____
- ☐ _____
- ☐ _____
- ☐ _____

NUTS
- ☐ almonds
- ☐ peanuts
- ☐ cashews
- ☐ walnuts
- ☐ pumpkin seeds
- ☐ flax seeds
- ☐ nut butter
  (peanut, almond etc)
- ☐ _____

BEANS
- ☐ black beans
- ☐ garbanzo beans
- ☐ hummus
- ☐ kidney beans
- ☐ navy beans
- ☐ pinto beans
- ☐ soy milk
- ☐ tofu
- ☐ _____
- ☐ _____
- ☐ _____

WHOLE GRAINS
- ☐ brown rice
- ☐ forbidden rice
- ☐ wild rice
- ☐ quinoa
- ☐ wheat bread
- ☐ couscous
- ☐ wheat pasta
- ☐ oatmeal
- ☐ _____
- ☐ _____

OTHER STUFF
- ☐ _____
- ☐ _____
- ☐ _____
- ☐ _____

DAIRY
- ☐ Cheese
- ☐ plain yogurt
- ☐ cow milk
- ☐ _____
- ☐ _____
- ☐ _____

LEAN PROTEIN
- ☐ eggs
- ☐ chicken
- ☐ turkey
- ☐ fish
- ☐ almond milk
- ☐ protein powder
- ☐ _____
- ☐ _____
- ☐ _____

GOOD FATS
- ☐ olive oil
- ☐ butter
- ☐ _____
- ☐ _____
- ☐ _____

DON'T FORGET
- ☐ _____
- ☐ _____
- ☐ _____
- ☐ _____

Week: _____   Date: _____

Sleep Metrics	Exercise Matters	Food Score	Meal Log
Monday			
Sleep estimate: _____ continuous/uninterrupted Quality: _____ Time I got in bed: _____ Time I woke up: _____ What made sleep better? _____ What made sleep worse? _____ Menses day: _____	Run-walk (min): _____ Distance: _____ Weather: _____ Ache, pain, or injury: _____ Treatments: _____ Steps: _____	Veggies (4): _____ Fruits(3): _____ Beans (1-2): _____ Protein (1-2): _____ Nuts (0.5): _____ Grains (2): _____ Good fats: _____ Dairy (1): _____ Quality points: _____ Deductions: _____ Food score: _____	BG: Fasting: _____ Two hours after meal: _____ Breakfast AM snack Lunch PM snack Dinner
Tuesday			
Sleep estimate: _____ continuous/uninterrupted Quality: _____ Time I got in bed: _____ Time I woke up: _____ What made sleep better? _____ What made sleep worse? _____ Menses day: _____	Run-walk (min): _____ Distance: _____ Weather: _____ Ache, pain, or injury: _____ Treatments: _____ Steps: _____	Veggies (4): _____ Fruits(3): _____ Beans (1-2): _____ Protein (1-2): _____ Nuts (0.5): _____ Grains (2): _____ Good fats: _____ Dairy (1): _____ Quality points: _____ Deductions: _____ Food score: _____	BG: Fasting: _____ Two hours after meal: _____ Breakfast AM snack Lunch PM snack Dinner

Wednesday

Sleep estimate: ____
continuous/uninterrupted
Quality: ____
Time I got in bed: ____
Time I woke up: ____
What made sleep better? ____
What made sleep worse? ____
Menses day: ____

Run-walk (min): ____
Distance: ____
Weather: ____
Ache, pain, or injury: ____
Treatments: ____
Steps: ____

Veggies (4): ____
Fruits(3): ____
Beans (1-2): ____
Protein (1-2): ____
Nuts (0.5): ____
Grains (2): ____
Good fats: ____
Dairy (1): ____
Quality points: ____
Deductions: ____
Food score: ____

BG: Fasting: ____
Two hours after meal: ____
Breakfast
AM snack
Lunch
PM snack
Dinner

Thursday

Sleep estimate: ____
continuous/uninterrupted
Quality: ____
Time I got in bed: ____
Time I woke up: ____
What made sleep better? ____
What made sleep worse? ____
Menses day: ____

Run-walk (min): ____
Distance: ____
Weather: ____
Ache, pain, or injury: ____
Treatments: ____
Steps: ____

Veggies (4): ____
Fruits(3): ____
Beans (1-2): ____
Protein (1-2): ____
Nuts (0.5): ____
Grains (2): ____
Good fats: ____
Dairy (1): ____
Quality points: ____
Deductions: ____
Food score: ____

BG: Fasting: ____
Two hours after meal: ____
Breakfast
AM snack
Lunch
PM snack
Dinner

Report Card

Tally for the Week	Health Numbers	Reflections
Days I met my run-walk goal: ___ Total miles: ___ Days my food score was ≥6: ___	Weight: ___ Body fat %: ___ Waist: ___ BP: ___ / ___ Resting heart rate: ___ Fasting blood sugar: ___	I feel... What works well for me?

Friday

	Health Numbers	Reflections
Sleep estimate: ___ continuous/ uninterrupted Quality: ___ Time I got in bed: ___ Time I woke up: ___ What made sleep better? What made sleep worse? Menses day: ___	Run-walk (min): ___ Distance: ___ Weather: ___ Ache, pain, or injury: Treatments: ___ Steps: ___	Veggies (4): ___ Fruits(3): ___ Beans (1-2): ___ Protein (1-2): ___ Nuts (0.5): ___ Grains (2): ___ Good fats: ___ Dairy (1): ___ Quality points: ___ Deductions: ___ Food score: ___ BG: Fasting: ___ Two hours after meal: ___ Breakfast AM snack Lunch PM snack Dinner

Saturday

Sleep estimate: _____ continuous/
uninterrupted
Quality: _____
Time I got in bed: _____
Time I woke up: _____
What made sleep better? _____
What made sleep worse? _____
Menses day: _____

Run-walk (min): _____
Distance: _____
Weather: _____
Ache, pain, or injury: _____
Treatments: _____
Steps: _____

Veggies (4): _____
Fruits(3): _____
Beans (1-2): _____
Protein (1-2): _____
Nuts (0.5): _____
Grains (2): _____
Good fats: _____
Dairy (1): _____
Quality points: _____
Deductions: _____
Food score: _____

BG: Fasting: _____
Two hours after meal: _____
Breakfast
AM snack
Lunch
PM snack
Dinner

Sunday

Sleep estimate: _____ continuous/
uninterrupted
Quality: _____
Time I got in bed: _____
Time I woke up: _____
What made sleep better? _____
What made sleep worse? _____
Menses day: _____

Run-walk (min): _____
Distance: _____
Weather: _____
Ache, pain, or injury: _____
Treatments: _____
Steps: _____

Veggies (4): _____
Fruits(3): _____
Beans (1-2): _____
Protein (1-2): _____
Nuts (0.5): _____
Grains (2): _____
Good fats: _____
Dairy (1): _____
Quality points: _____
Deductions: _____
Food score: _____

BG: Fasting: _____
Two hours after meal: _____
Breakfast
AM snack
Lunch
PM snack
Dinner

CREDITS

Design and Layout

Cover Design: Katerina Georgieva
Cover Photo: ©AdobeStock
Interior Design: Annika Naas
Layout: Angela K. Snyder

Editorial

Managing Editor: Elizabeth Evans
Copyeditor: Anne Rumery

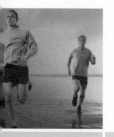

THE ESSENTIAL JEFF GALLOWAY

All information subject to change © Adobe Stock

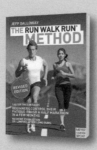

1st reprint
192 p., color, paperback,
16,5 x 24,0 cm
ISBN: 9781782550822
$18.95 US

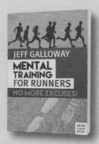

3rd edition
208 p., color, paperback,
16,5 x 24,0 cm
ISBN: 9781782550839
$18.95 US

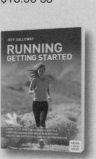

1st reprint of the 5th edition
240 p., color, paperback,
16,5 x 24,0 cm
ISBN: 9781782550549
$16.95 US

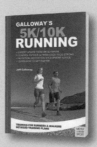

1st reprint of the 3rd edition
200 p., color, paperback,
5.5" x 8.5"
ISBN: 9781841263366
$16.95 US

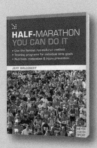

5th edition
216 p., color, paperback,
16,5 x 24,0 cm
ISBN: 9781841263335
$16.95 US

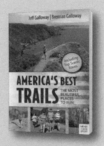

revised
304 p., color, paperback,
16,5 x 24,0 cm
ISBN: 978-1-78255-096-9
$18.95 US

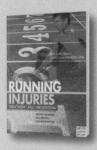

1st reprint of the first edition
168 p., color, paperback,
16,5 x 24,0 cm
ISBN: 9781841262840
$16.95 US

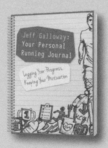

184 p., color, Spiral bound,
14,8 x 21 cm
ISBN: 9781782551102
$15.95 US

MEYER & MEYER Sport
Von-Coels-Str. 390
52080 Aachen
Germany

Phone   +49 02 41 - 9 58 10 - 13
Fax   +49 02 41 - 9 58 10 - 10
E-Mail   sales@m-m-sports.com
E-Books   www.m-m-sports.com

All books available as E-books.

MEYER
& MEYER
SPORT

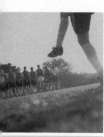

THE ROAD IS THE GOAL

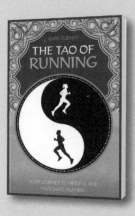

304 p., b/w, paperback,
45 photos
5.5" x 8.5"
ISBN: 9781782550754
$13.95 US

All information subject to change © Adobe Stock

Gary Dudney

THE TAO OF RUNNING
YOUR JOURNEY TO MINDFUL
AND PASSIONATE RUNNING

Running is more than moving one foot in front of the other. Running can evoke spiritualism and mindfulness; it can teach fundamental lessons about goals, self-awareness, and self-improvement; it can be a transformative existential experience. *The Tao of Running* offers a fresh perspective on this mental side of running while entertaining with vivid tales of running adventures. Going well beyond the standard training and racing advice found in most running books, it guides runners to a wider understanding of how running fits into their own aspirations, goals, and life philosophy. Readers will gain a greater appreciation for the rewards and possibilities inherent in running and will significantly deepen, enlighten, and enrich their running experience.

GET RID OF CELLULITE!

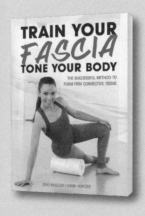

200 p., color, paperback,
120 photos
16,5 x 24,0 cm
ISBN: 9781782551171
$13.95 US

Gary Dudney

TRAIN YOUR FASCIA, TONE YOUR BODY
THE SUCCESSFUL METHOD TO FORM FIRM CONNECTIVE TISSUE

Fascia is a building network in our body that gives us support, structure, and form. Whether a thigh is firm and beautifully shaped or like jelly depends on the tone of the fibrous connective tissue—the fascia. Therefore, we must train and firm the fascia in addition to strengthening the muscles. Only then will we have defined muscles, a well-toned body contour, and a slender shape. In collaboration with renowned fascia researcher, Robert Schleip, PhD, Divo Müller has developed new training that specifically tones connective tissue. Applying the power principles presented in the illustrated and detailed full-body workouts—sense, bounce, tone, and nourish—you can reduce cellulite and eliminate bat wings and a flabby bottom.

MEYER & MEYER Sport
Von-Coels-Str. 390
52080 Aachen
Germany

Phone	+49 02 41 - 9 58 10 - 13
Fax	+49 02 41 - 9 58 10 - 10
E-Mail	sales@m-m-sports.com
E-Books	www.m-m-sports.com

All books available as E-books.

MEYER
& MEYER
SPORT